Essential
to Acute Care

Nicola Cooper

Specialist Registrar in General Internal Medicine and Care of the Elderly, Yorkshire, UK

Paul Cramp

Consultant in Anaesthesia and Intensive Care, Bradford Teaching Hospitals NHS Trust, UK

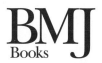

First published in 2003
by BMJ Books, BMA House, Tavistock Square,
London WC1H 9JR

Reprinted 2004

www.bmjbooks.com

British Library Cataloguing in Publication Data

A catalogue record for this book is available from the British Library
ISBN 0 7279 1648 3

Typeset by SIVA Math Setters, Chennai, India
Printed and bound in Spain by GraphyCems, Navarra

Contents

Introduction

'...in the beginning of the malady it is easy to cure but difficult to detect, but in the course of time, not having been either detected or treated ... it becomes easy to detect but difficult to cure.'

Niccolo Machiavelli, *The Prince*

This book is aimed at trainees in internal medicine, surgery, anaesthesia, intensive care, and emergency medicine – people who deal with acutely ill adults. Final year medical students and nursing staff in critical care areas will also find this book extremely useful.

There are many books on the management of patients who are acutely ill, but all have a traditional "recipe" format. One looks up a diagnosis and the management is summarised. Few of us are trained how to deal with the generic altered physiology that can accompany acute illness. The result is that many doctors are unable to deal logically with patients in physiological decline and this often leads to suboptimal care.

In our surveys of doctors of all specialties, few can explain how different oxygen masks work, the difference between hypercapnic respiratory failure and "CO_2 retention", what a fluid challenge is and how to effectively treat organ failure.

This book contains information that you really need to know and that is not found in a standard textbook. Throughout the text are "mini-tutorials" that explain the latest thinking or controversies. Case histories and problem-solving exercises are included at the end of each chapter. Further reading is included for more information. It is our aim that this book should provide a foundation in learning how to care effectively for those who are acutely ill.

Nicola Cooper and Paul Cramp

Units used in this book

Standard International (SI) units are used throughout this book, with metric units in brackets where these differ. Below are some reference ranges for common blood results. Reference ranges vary from laboratory to laboratory.

Metric units × conversion factor = SI units

Test	Metric units	Conversion factor	SI units
Sodium	135–145 meq/litre	1	135–145 mmol/litre
Potassium	3·5–5·0 meq/litre	1	3·5–5·0 mmol/litre
Urea (blood urea nitrogen)	8–20 mg/dl	0·36	2·9–7·1 mmol/litre
Creatinine	0·6–1·2 mg/dl	83·3	50–100 µmol/litre
Glucose	60–115 mg/dl	0·06	3·3–6·3 mmol/litre
Partial pressure O_2	83–108 mmHg	0·13	11–14·36 kPa
Partial pressure CO_2	32–48 mmHg	0·13	4·26–6·38 kPa
Bicarbonate	22–28 meq/litre	1	22–28 mmol/litre
Calcium	8·5–10·5 mg/dl	0·25	2·1–2·6 mmol/litre
Chloride	98–107 meq/litre	1	98–107 mmol/litre
Lactate	0·5–2·0 meq/litre	1	0·5–2·0 mmol/litre

Abbreviations

Please find below a list of common abbreviations used throughout this book.

ACTH adrenocorticotropic hormone
ADH antidiuretic hormone
AF atrial fibrillation
ALI acute lung injury
APC activated protein C
ARDS acute respiratory distress syndrome
ARF acute renal failure
AS aortic stenosis
ATLS Advanced Trauma and Life Support
ATN acute tubular necrosis
BE base excess
BiPAP biphasic or bilevel positive airway pressure
BP blood pressure
BUN blood urea nitrogen
CAVH continuous arteriovenous haemofiltration
CBF cerebral blood flow
CO cardiac output
COPD chronic obstructive pulmonary disease
CPAP continuous positive airway pressure
CPP cerebral perfusion pressure
CPR cardiopulmonary resuscitation
CT computed tomography
CVP central venous pressure
CVVH continuous venovenous haemofiltration
DIC disseminated intravascular coagulation
DO_2 oxygen delivery
DVT deep vein thrombosis
ECF extracellular fluid

EFW electrolyte-free water

ERCP endoscopic retrograde cholangiopancreatogram

FiO_2 fraction of inspired oxygen

FVC forced vital capacity

GCS Glasgow Coma Scale

Hb haemoglobin

HDUs high dependency units

HES hydroxyethyl starch

HR heart rate

ICF intracellular fluid

ICP intracranial pressure

ICU Intensive Care Unit

IPPV intermittent positive pressure ventilation

LIDCO lithium dilution and arterial waveform analysis

LP lumbar puncture

LVEDP left ventricular end-diastolic pressure

MAP mean arterial pressure

METs medical emergency teams

METS metabolic equivalents

MODS multiple organ dysfunction syndrome

MRI magnetic resonance imaging

MRSA methicillin-resistant *Staphylococcus aureus*

NIV non-invasive ventilation

NSAIDs non-steroidal anti-inflammatory drugs

OSA obstructive sleep apnoea

PAF platelet-activating factor

PAO_2 or $PACO_2$ alveolar partial pressure of oxygen or carbon dioxide

PaO_2 or $PaCO_2$ arterial partial pressure of oxygen or carbon dioxide

PAOP pulmonary artery occlusion pressure

PE pulmonary embolism

PEEP positive end-expiratory pressure

PiCCO transpulmonary thermodilution and arterial pulse contour analysis

PSV pressure support ventilation

RRT renal replacement therapy

SAH subarachnoid haemorrhage

SaO_2 arterial oxygen saturation of haemoglobin

SID strong ion difference

SIMV synchronised intermittent mandatory ventilation

SIRS systemic inflammatory response syndrome

SV stroke volume

SVR systemic vascular resistance

SVRI systemic vascular resistance index

TBI traumatic brain injury

TBW total body water

TF tissue factor

TNF tumour necrosis factor

TTP thrombotic thrombocytopenic purpura

1: Patients at risk

By the end of this chapter you will be able to:
- redefine resuscitation
- recognise patients at risk and understand early warning scores
- know about current developments in this area
- understand the importance of the generic altered physiology that accompanies acute illness (understanding A, B, C, D)
- know how to communicate effectively with colleagues
- understand the benefits and limitations of intensive care
- have a context for the chapters that follow

Redefining resuscitation

Cardiopulmonary resuscitation (CPR) has evolved over the last 40 years into a significant part of healthcare training. International organisations govern resuscitation protocols. Yet survival to discharge after in-hospital CPR is poor. Study survival rates range from 2 to 14%. Public perception of CPR is informed by television where there are far better outcomes than in reality.

A great deal of attention is focused on saving life after cardiac arrest, but the vast majority of in-hospital cardiac arrests are predictable. Hardly any attention is focused on detecting commonplace reversible physiological deterioration or preventing cardiac arrest in the first place. Two studies illustrate this well. In 1990, Schein *et al.* found that 84% of patients had documented observations of clinical deterioration or new complaints within 8 hours of arrest; 70% had either deterioration of respiratory or mental function observed during this time. Whilst there did not appear to be any single reproducible warning signs, the average respiratory rate of the patients prior to arrest was 30 per minute. The investigators observed that the predominantly respiratory and metabolic derangements which preceded cardiac arrest (hypoxaemia, hypotension, and acidosis) were not rapidly fatal and that efforts to predict and prevent arrest would therefore be beneficial. Only 8% patients survived to discharge after CPR in this study. In 1994, Franklin *et al.* observed that documented

---

Box 1.1 Recognition of critical illness

1. Physiological
   - Signs of massive sympathetic activation, for example, raised heart rate, blood pressure, pale, shut down
   - Signs of systemic inflammation (see chapter 7)
   - Signs of organ hypoperfusion, for example, cold peripheries, increased respiratory rate, oliguria (see chapter 5)

2. Biochemical
   - Base deficit/raised lactate
   - Raised or low white cell count
   - Low platelets
   - Raised urea and creatinine
   - Raised CRP

---

physiological deterioration occurred within 6 hours in 66% of patients with cardiac arrest, but no action was taken.

Researchers have commented that there appears to be a failure of the system to recognise and effectively intervene when patients in hospital deteriorate. There is little postgraduate training in the resuscitation of critically ill adults (that is, A, B, C, D – airway, breathing, circulation and disability), and in the UK there are too few available senior staff who have the skills to manage these patients effectively. This impacts on the quality of admissions to the Intensive Care Unit (ICU). In 1999, McGloin *et al.* observed that 36% ICU admissions received suboptimal care beforehand and that survival was worse in this group. In 1998 McQuillan *et al.* looked at 100 emergency ICU admissions. Two external assessors observed that only 20 cases were well managed beforehand. The majority (54) received suboptimal care prior to admission to ICU and there was disagreement over the remaining 26 cases. The patients were of a similar case-mix and APACHE II (acute physiological and chronic health evaluation) scores. In the suboptimal group, ICU admission was considered late in 69% cases and avoidable altogether in 41%. The main causes of suboptimal care were considered to be failure of organisation, lack of knowledge, failure to appreciate the clinical urgency, lack of supervision, and failure to seek advice. Other studies have shown that suboptimal care before admission to ICU increases mortality by around 50%. ICU mortality is doubled if the patient is admitted from a general ward rather than from theatres or the Emergency Department, in theory because they arrive so sick that they are unlikely to recover.

Resuscitation is therefore not about CPR. It is about recognising patients in physiological decline in the first place and then effectively treating them. This is an area of medicine that has been neglected in terms of training, organisation, and resources.

Medical emergency teams

Ken Hillman first developed medical emergency teams (METs) in Sydney, Australia as an alternative to the cardiac arrest team. The MET was alerted to any critical changes in A, B, C or D and parameters were provided for guidance. The MET included an ICU doctor and an ICU nurse. At its disposal was a critical care facility larger than in most UK hospitals.

In Liverpool, UK, there has been a rise in the number of MET calls (up to 44% occurring at night) since it was formed and a decline in the number of cardiac arrests. This is due to an increase in "Do not attempt CPR" orders as well as prevention of cardiac arrests: 25% patients seen by the MET were deemed to be unsuitable for CPR, although that decision had not yet been made by the referring team. General wards in the UK are increasingly likely to be filled with patients at risk of physiological decline. Most patients admitted to ICU have obvious physiological derangements (Figure 1.1). They are recognised by general ward staff as being at risk, yet there is often a lack of effective intervention.

Up to 30% patients admitted to ICUs in the UK have had a cardiac or respiratory arrest in the preceding 24 hours. Most of these are already hospital in-patients. Half die immediately and mortality for the rest on ICU is at least 70%. The purpose of a medical emergency team instead of a cardiac arrest team is simple – early action saves lives. As Peter Safar, a pioneer of resuscitation, has commented, "the most sophisticated intensive care often becomes unnecessarily expensive terminal care when the pre-ICU system fails".

Current developments

In October 1999, the publication in the UK of the Audit Commission's *Critical to Success – the place of efficient and*

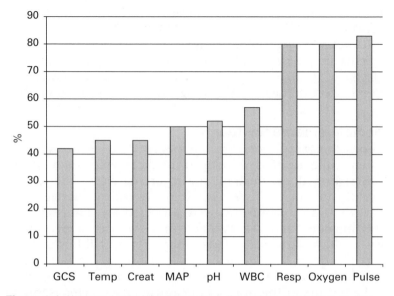

Figure 1.1 Abnormal physiological values (%) before admission to ICU. Reproduced with permission from Theta Press Ltd (Goldhill D. Medical Emergency Teams. *Care of the Critically Ill*. 2000;**16**:209–12. Creat, creatinine; GCS, Glasgow Coma Score; MAP, mean arterial pressure; Resp, respiratory rate; Temp, temperature, WBC, white blood cells

effective critical care services within the acute hospital re-emphasised the concept of the patient at risk – patients at risk of their condition deteriorating into a need for critical care. The report advocated better training of medical and nursing staff, early warning scoring systems and "outreach" critical care. The Commission commented that intensive care is something that tends to happen within four walls, but that patients should not be defined by what bed they occupy, but by their severity of illness (Box 1.2).

Following this, *Comprehensive Critical Care – a review of adult critical care services* was published by the Department of Health. The report reiterated the idea that patients should be classified according to their severity of illness and the necessary resources mobilised. This includes critical care outreach teams. In the USA and parts of Europe, there is considerable provision of high dependency units (HDUs). In most UK hospitals it is recognised that there are not enough HDU facilities. A needs assessment survey in Wales, using

Box 1.2 New UK severity of illness classification

- Level 0: Patients whose needs can be met through normal ward care in an acute hospital

- Level 1: Patients at risk of their condition deteriorating, or those recently relocated from higher levels of care, whose needs can be met on an acute ward with additional advice and support from the critical care team

- Level 2: Patients requiring more detailed observation or intervention including support for a single failing organ system or post-operative care and those 'stepping down' from higher levels of care

- Level 3: Patients requiring advanced respiratory support alone or basic respiratory support together with support of at least two organ systems. This level includes all complex patients requiring support for multi-organ failure

Level 2 is equivalent to previous HDU care; Level 3 is equivalent to previous ICU care. Reproduced with permission from DOH (*Comprehensive critical care*. London, Department of Health, 2000).

objective criteria for HDU and ICU admission, found that 56% of these patients were being cared for on general wards rather than in critical care areas. A 1-month needs assessment in Newcastle, UK found that 26% of the unselected emergency patients admitted to a medical admissions unit required a higher level of care: 17% needed level 1 care, 9% needed level 2 care and 0·5% level 2 care. This would indicate the need for far higher level 1–2 facilities in the UK than at present.

Early warning scores have been developed and advocated as a means of targeting resources early and therefore more effectively (Table 1.1). Increasingly abnormal vital signs mean that the patient is sick and a high score requires early assessment and intervention by experienced staff. Whilst these scores could lead to a false sense of security if they are normal, evidence is emerging that early warning scores can reduce CPR rates and ICU mortality (Figure 1.2).

A, B, C, D – an overview

History, examination, differential diagnosis and treatment will not help someone who is critically ill. Diagnosis is

Table 1.1 An example early warning scoring system.

Score	3	2	1	0	1	2	3
Heart rate		< 40	41–50	51–100	101–110	111–130	> 130
Systolic BP	< 70	71–80	81–100	101–179	180–199	200–220	> 220
Respiratory rate		< 8	8–11	12–20	21–25	26–30	> 30
Conscious level			Confused	A	V	P	U
Urine (ml/4 h)	< 80	80–120	120–200		> 800		
O_2 saturations	< 85%	86–89%	90–94%	> 95%			
O_2 therapy	NIV or CPAP	> 60% oxygen	O_2 therapy				

Each observation has a score. If the total score is 4 or more (the cut-off varies between institutions), a doctor is called to assess the patient.

NIV, non-invasive ventilation; CPAP, non-invasive continuous positive airway pressure; A, alert; V, responds to verbal commands; P, responds to painful stimuli; U, unresponsive.

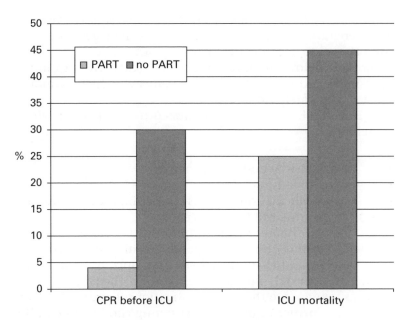

Figure 1.2 Impact of PART in a London hospital. Abbreviations: CPR, cardiopulmonary resuscitation; ICU, intensive care unit; PART, patient at risk team. Reproduced with permission from Theta Press Ltd (Goldhill D. Medical Emergency Teams. *Care of the Critically Ill*. 2000;**16**:209–12

irrelevant when the things that kill first are literally A (airway compromise), B (breathing problems), and C (circulation problems) – in that order. What the patient needs is resuscitation not deliberation. Patients can be alert and "look" well from the end of the bed, but the clue is often in the vital signs. A common theme in studies is the inability of hospital staff to recognise when a patient is at risk. Even when the vital signs are documented, there is a failure to appreciate that serious abnormal physiology is an emergency.

The most common abnormalities before cardiac arrest are hypoxaemia with an increased respiratory rate and hypotension leading to hypoperfusion with an accompanying metabolic acidosis and tissue hypoxia. Hypoperfusion is common in hospital. If this is left untreated, a downward physiological spiral ensues. With time the hypoperfusion may become resistant to treatment with fluids and drugs. Therefore early action is vital. The following chapters teach the theory behind A, B, C, D in detail. Practical courses also exist that use scenario-based teaching on how to manage patients at risk. These are recommended because the A, B, C approach described below requires practical skills (for example, assessment and management of the airway), which cannot be learned adequately from a book.

A, B, C, D, E is the initial approach to any patient who is acutely ill:

- **A** – assess airway and treat if needed
- **B** – assess breathing and treat if needed
- **C** – assess circulation (that is, pulse, blood pressure, and skin perfusion) and treat if needed
- **D** – assess disability (the simple AVPU scale can be used (alert, responds to voice, responds to pain, unresponsive)
- **E** – expose and examine patient fully once A, B, and C are stable. Arterial blood gases and a bedside glucose measurement are the first investigations in any critically ill patient. Further information gathering can be done at this stage – for example, further history and details from notes and charts.

If there is one thing in medicine which is evidence-based, it is that patients with serious abnormal physiology are an emergency. The management of such patients requires pro-activity, a sense of urgency, and the continuous presence of the attending doctor. For example, if a patient is hypotensive and hypoxaemic from pneumonia, it is not acceptable for oxygen, fluids, and antibiotics simply to be prescribed. The oxygen concentration may need to be changed several times before the PaO_2 is acceptable. More than one fluid challenge may be required to get an acceptable blood pressure – and even then, vasopressors may be needed if the patient remains hypotensive because of severe sepsis. Intravenous antibiotics need to be given immediately. ICU and CPR decisions need to be made at this time – not later. The emphasis is on both rapid and effective intervention.

Integral to the management of the acutely ill patient is the administration of effective analgesia. This is not discussed further in subsequent chapters but it is extremely important. Suffice to say that titrated intravenous analgesia is the method of choice in critically ill patients who suffer from delayed gastric emptying and reduced skin and muscle perfusion, making oral, subcutaneous, or intramuscular drugs less reliable.

Communication and the critically ill

A new doctor once asked his senior how to treat a patient who had too much beta blocker. The senior was half listening, writing in some notes. Another senior was nearby and asked, "What do you mean – what is the pulse and blood pressure?" The new doctor replied, "Pulse 30, blood pressure unrecordable". Both seniors dashed to the patient's bedside. It is important to communicate well if you want other people to act. When talking to a colleague about a patient who is acutely ill, use the following guide:

* where you are and your request (for example, "Can you come to ...?")
* brief history (for example, "New admission with asthma") and current physiology: conscious level, pulse, blood pressure, respiratory rate, oxygen saturations (and urine output if relevant)
* further details can follow (for example, test results).

It is important to give a summary of the current physiology, which gives the listener a sense of how urgent the case is. It is also important to communicate clearly what help is needed, particularly if you want your colleague to come and see the patient.

The benefits and limitations of intensive care

Physiological derangement and the need for admission to ICU is not the same thing. It would not be in the best interests of all patients to be admitted to an ICU; instead optimising ward care or even palliative care may be required. Intensive care supports failing organ systems when there is potentially reversible disease. Intensive (level 3) care is appropriate for patients requiring advanced respiratory support alone or support of at least two failing organ systems. High dependency (level 2) care is appropriate for patients requiring detailed observation or intervention for a single failing organ system. For the majority of people who have never worked in an ICU, the benefits and limitations of what is available may be poorly understood. Patients with acute reversible disease benefit most from intensive care if they are admitted sooner rather than later. Waiting for someone to become even more critically ill before contacting the ICU team is not evidence-based. On the other hand, some patients may be so ill they are unlikely to recover at all – even with intensive organ support. All potential admissions should therefore be assessed by an experienced doctor. Patients who are not admitted to the ICU can (and should) still receive good ward care.

The following chapters will describe the theory behind the assessment and management of acutely ill adults. They are intended as a foundation upon which experience and practical training can be built. Understanding and practising the basics well can prevent in-hospital deaths and admissions to ICU.

Further reading

Audit Commission. *Critical to success – the place of efficient and effective critical care services within the acute hospital.* London: Audit Commission, 1999.

Department of Health. *Comprehensive Critical Care – a review of adult critical care services.* London: DoH, 2000.

Franklin C, Matthew J. Developing strategies to prevent in-hospital cardiac arrest: analysing responses to physicians and nurses in the hourse before the event. *Crit Care Med* 1994;**22**:244–7.

Goldhill D. Medical Emergency Teams. *Care of the Critically Ill* 2000;**16**: 209–12.

Hillman K, Parr M, Flabouris A, Bishop G, Stewart A. Redefining in-hospital resuscitation: the concept of the medical emergency team. *Resuscitation* 2001;**48**:105–10.

McGloin H, Adam SK, Singer M. Unexpected deaths and referrals to Intensive Care of patient on general wards: are some potentially avoidable? *J R Coll Physicians* 1999;**33**:255–9.

McQuillan P, Pilkington S, Allan A *et al.* Confidential enquiry into quality of care before admission to intensive care. *BMJ* 1998;**316**:1853–8.

Royal College of Physicians of London. *Working party report on the interface between acute general [internal] medicine and critical care.* London: RCPL, 2002.

Schein RM, Hazday N, Pena N, Ruben BH. Clinical antecedents to in-hospital cardiopulmonary arrest. *Chest* 1990;**98**:1388–92.

Practical courses on the management of acutely ill adults

ALERT (acute life-threatening events recognition and treatment). A generic acute care course developed by the School of Postgraduate Medicine, University of Portsmouth, UK.

CCrIMP (care of the critically ill medical patient) is being developed with the Royal College of Physicians of London.

CCrISP (care of the critically ill surgical patient) is run by the Royal College of Surgeons of England and Edinburgh.

ALS (advanced life support) is run by the Resuscitation Council UK. This course centres on the management of cardiac arrest and peri-arrest scenarios.

ATLS (advanced trauma and life support) is run by the Royal College of Surgeons of England and Edinburgh and focuses on trauma care.

2: Oxygen

By the end of this chapter you will be able to:
- understand how to prescribe oxygen therapy
- understand what hypoxaemia is
- understand the different devices used to deliver oxygen
- optimise oxygen delivery
- understand the limitations of pulse oximetry
- understand the difference between "CO_2 retention" from uncontrolled oxygen therapy and hypercapnic respiratory failure owing to other reasons
- apply this to your clinical practice

Myths about oxygen

Oxygen was discovered by Joseph Priestley in 1777 and has become one of the most commonly used drugs in medical practice. Yet it is poorly prescribed by most medical staff. In 2000 we carried out two surveys of oxygen therapy. The first looked at oxygen prescriptions in postoperative patients in a large district general hospital. It found that there were several dozen ways used to prescribe oxygen and that the prescriptions were rarely followed. The second surveyed 50 medical and nursing staff working on a medical admissions, coronary care, and respiratory unit of another district hospital. They were asked questions about oxygen masks and the concentration of oxygen delivered by each mask. They were also asked which mask was most appropriate for a range of clinical situations and how much oxygen may be given to patients with chronic obstructive pulmonary disease (COPD). The answers were very revealing:

- Many people could not name the different types of oxygen mask.
- The relationship between litres per minute and oxygen concentration (%) was poorly understood – for example, most people thought that a patient receives 28% oxygen from nasal cannulae at 2 litres per minute and 100% oxygen from a mask with a reservoir bag at 15 litres per minute.

- One-third chose a 28% Venturi mask for an unwell patient with asthma.
- Just over one-third thought that a diagnosis of COPD meant that one could never give more than 28% oxygen.
- Not one person understood the different reasons why $PaCO_2$ rises – the difference between "CO_2 retention" from uncontrolled oxygen therapy and hypercapnic respiratory failure owing to other causes. Reducing the oxygen concentration in order to "treat" a high $PaCO_2$ was common practice.
- It was common practice to use simple face masks at 2 litres per minute if the patient had COPD.

There are many false beliefs about oxygen and the result is that many patients are incorrectly treated. Yet oxygen is a drug with a correct concentration and side effects.

Hypoxaemia

Hypoxaemia is defined as the reduction below normal levels of oxygen in arterial blood – a PaO_2 of < 8·0 kPa (60 mmHg) or oxygen saturations < 90%. Hypoxia is the reduction below normal levels of oxygen in the tissues. The normal range for arterial blood oxygen is 11–14 kPa (85–105 mmHg), which reduces in old age. It is hypoxia rather than hypoxaemia that causes cell damage. Hypoxaemia usually results in hypoxia.

The main causes of hypoxaemia are:

- ventilation–perfusion ($\dot{V}/\dot{Q}$) mismatch
- intrapulmonary shunt
- hypoventilation
- increased oxygen consumption.

Severe tissue hypoxia results in cell death and organ damage. In the ward setting, simple oxygen therapy may reverse the confusion, agitation, and cardiac ischaemia that is seen in such circumstances.

Oxygen therapy

There are very few formal criteria for the use of oxygen in hospital. The American College of Chest Physicians and the

National Heart, Lung and Blood Institute has published the following recommendations for instituting oxygen therapy:

* cardiorespiratory arrest
* hypoxaemia (PaO_2 < 8·0 kPa/60 mmHg or saturations < 90%)
* hypotension (systolic blood pressure < 100 mmHg)
* low cardiac output with metabolic acidosis
* respiratory distress (respiratory rate > 24 per minute).

Oxygen is also indicated in the perioperative period, in trauma or other acute illness, carbon monoxide poisoning, severe anaemia, and when drugs are used that may reduce ventilation, such as opioids.

In general, the devices available to deliver oxygen can be split into two categories depending on whether they deliver a proportion of, or the entire, ventilatory requirement (Figure 2.1; Table 2.1):

* Low flow devices deliver oxygen at less than the inspiratory flow rate, for example nasal cannulae and simple face masks (including masks with a reservoir bag). Although they are low flow, they can deliver a high concentration of oxygen. The oxygen concentration is variable.
* High flow devices deliver oxygen at above the inspiratory flow rate, such as Venturi masks. Although they are high flow, a low concentration of oxygen may be delivered. The oxygen concentration is fixed.

Low flow devices – nasal cannulae, simple face masks and reservoir bag masks

Nasal cannulae are commonly used because they are convenient and comfortable. They deliver 2–4 litres per minute of 100% oxygen in addition to the air a person is breathing. If a person is breathing slowly with 10 breaths per minute and 500 ml tidal volumes, the minute volume (or inspiratory flow rate) will be only 5 litres per minute. So the patient receives 2 litres per minute of 100% oxygen plus 3 litres per minute of air. Two-fifths of what the patient is breathing is 100% oxygen. However, a person breathing quickly (40 breaths per minute and 750 ml tidal volumes) will

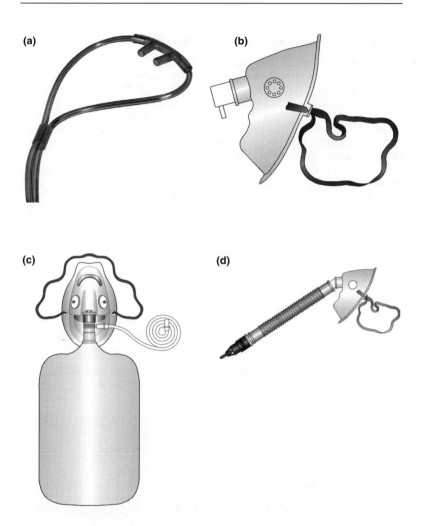

Venturi valve colour	Flow rate (litres per minute)	Concentration (%)
Blue	2	24
White	4	28
Yellow	6	35
Red	8	40
Green	12	60

Figure 2.1 Different oxygen masks. (a) Nasal cannulae; (b) simple face mask; (c) reservoir bag mask; (d) Venturi mask. Reproduced with permission from Intersurgical Complete Respiratory Systems, Wokingham, Berkshire

Table 2.1 Which mask for which patient?

Oxygen device	Patients
Nasal cannulae	Patients with otherwise normal physiology (vital signs), for example, postoperative, slightly low SaO_2, long-term oxygen therapy
Simple face masks and masks with reservoir bag (> 5 litres/min aiming for SaO_2 > 94%)	Higher concentrations required and controlled O_2 not necessary, for example, severe asthma, acute left ventricular failure, pneumonia, trauma, severe sepsis
Venturi masks	Controlled oxygen therapy required, for example, patients with COPD

have a minute volume of 30 litres per minute, so 2 litres per minute of 100% oxygen should be given plus 28 litres per minute air. Only two-thirtieths of what the patient is breathing is 100% oxygen. The person breathing slowly receives a large proportion of oxygen whilst the person breathing quickly receives much less. Thus nasal cannulae deliver a variable concentration of oxygen depending on how the patient is breathing. It is possible to estimate the concentration of oxygen by the calculations in Box 2.1.

Box 2.1 Calculation of oxygen concentration

- **Minute volume: 5 litres per minute** (for example, 10 breaths per minute × 500 ml per breath)
- **O_2 flow rate: 2 litres per minute**

Inspired O_2 concentration = 2 litres per minute of 100% O_2 + 3 litres per minute air

$$\frac{1 \times 2 + 0.21 \times 3}{5} = 53\%$$

- **Minute volume: 30 litres per minute** (for example, 40 breaths per minute × 750 ml/breath)
- **O_2 flow rate: 2 litres per minute**

Inspired O_2 concentration = 2 litres per minute of 100% O_2 + 28 litres per minute air

$$\frac{1 \times 2 + 0.21 \times 28}{30} = 26\%$$

In some cases the oxygen will not be enough and in some cases it could be dangerously high, for example in some patients who retain carbon dioxide. There are several case reports of these patients becoming unconscious with hypercapnia once they have been given nasal cannulae, especially during an acute exacerbation of their illness. There is no way of accurately knowing how much oxygen is being delivered.

Simple face masks (also called Hudson or MC masks) deliver up to 50% oxygen when set to 15 litres per minute. Like nasal cannulae, the concentration is variable depending on the fit of the mask and how the patient is breathing. Sometimes patients are given 2 litres per minute through face masks because they have COPD. Significant rebreathing of carbon dioxide can occur if the oxygen is set to < 5 litres per minute because exhaled air is not adequately flushed from the mask.

Face masks with a reservoir bag can deliver 70–80% oxygen at 15 litres per minute but this again depends on the fit of the mask and how the patient is breathing. A reservoir of oxygen is held in the bag. A non-rebreathe valve separates the bag and the mask so that the patient can inhale oxygen from it but not exhale back into it. Sometimes these masks are called "non rebreathe bag masks" for this reason. It is impossible for a patient to receive 100% oxygen via these masks for the simple reason that there is no air-tight seal between mask and patient. The reservoir bag should be filled with oxygen before the mask is placed on the patient. The bag should not deflate by more than two-thirds with each breath.

Nasal cannulae, simple face masks, and reservoir bag masks all deliver variable oxygen concentrations – or uncontrolled oxygen therapy.

High flow devices – Venturi masks

The Venturi valve increases the flow rate of oxygen and air to above the patient's inspiratory flow rate which is why these masks are more noisy (Figure 2.2). By doing this it can provide a constant oxygen concentration no matter how quickly or slowly the patient breathes. Venturi masks have colour-coded valves (labelled 24%, 28%, 35%, 40%, and 60%), which are

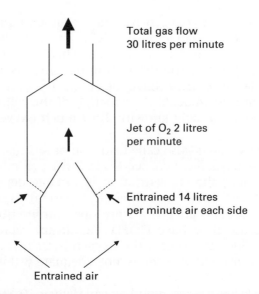

Total gas flow
30 litres per minute

Jet of O_2 2 litres
per minute

Entrained 14 litres
per minute air each side

Entrained air

Figure 2.2 Velocity or flow of gas in a Venturi mask. Bernoulli's equation for incompressible flow states that $0.5\ pv^2 + P = $ constant (where p is density), so, if the pressure (P) of a gas falls, it gains velocity (v). When gas moves through the Venturi valve, there is a sudden pressure drop, owing to the increase in area. The velocity or flow of the gas increases according to this equation

designed to deliver a fixed percentage of oxygen when set to the appropriate flow rate. To change the oxygen concentration, both the valve and flow have to be changed. At oxygen requirements over 40%, the mask may not have enough total flow to meet high inspiratory demands. Venturi masks are the mask of choice in acutely ill patients who require controlled oxygen therapy.

Flow is not the same as concentration. Low flow masks can deliver high concentrations of oxygen and high flow masks can deliver low concentrations of oxygen. Therefore the terms "high concentration" and "low concentration" are preferred when speaking about the amount of oxygen a patient is receiving. Humidified oxygen should be given when prolonged high concentrations are used as the airways may become dry. This impedes the expectoration of secretions, which can be extremely important in certain situations.

Oxygen delivery

Nearly all oxygen is carried to the tissues by haemoglobin (Hb). Each gram/dl of Hb carries 1·3 ml oxygen when fully saturated. A negligible amount is dissolved in plasma. The oxygen content of blood can therefore be calculated:

Hb (g/dl) × oxygen saturation of Hb × 1·3 and × 10 to convert to litres

The delivery of oxygen to the tissues depends on the cardiac output. From this we derive the oxygen delivery equation:

$$Hb \times SaO_2 \times 1{\cdot}3 \times 10 \times CO$$

Understanding that oxygen delivery depends on other factors as well as oxygen therapy will help to optimise oxygenation in any patient who is unwell. In a 70 kg man a normal Hb is 14 g/dl, normal saturation is above 95% and normal CO is 5 litres per minute. Oxygen delivery is therefore: 14 × 0·95 × 1·3 × 10 × 5 = 864·5 ml O_2 per minute. Patients with pneumonia or severe asthma can be extremely dehydrated. If a patient has an Hb of 14, an SaO_2 of 93%, and a reduced cardiac output (4 litres per minute) because of dehydration, his oxygen delivery is 14 × 0·93 × 1·3 × 10 × 4 = 677 ml O_2 per minute. By increasing his oxygen so that his saturations are now 98%, his oxygen delivery can be increased to 14 × 0·98 × 1·3 × 10 × 4 = 713 ml O_2 per minute, but if a fluid challenge is given to increase his cardiac output to normal (5 litres per minute) and his oxygen is kept the same, his oxygen delivery would be 14 × 0·93 × 1·3 × 10 × 5 = 846 ml O_2 per minute. Oxygen delivery has been increased more by giving fluid than by giving oxygen. The oxygen delivery equation also illustrates that an SaO_2 of 95% with severe anaemia is worse than an SaO_2 of 80% with a haemoglobin of 15 g/dl.

The oxygen-dissociation curve

Oxygen carriage in the blood relies on haemoglobin – the concentration, its carrying capacity and saturation. The percentage of Hb saturation with oxygen at different partial

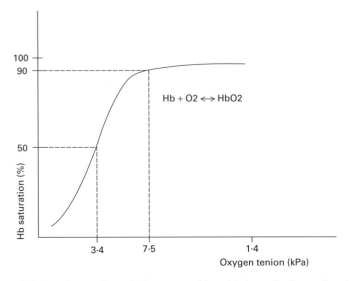

Figure 2.3 The oxygen-dissociation curve. Sigmoid shape is due to "positive cooperativity". Acidosis, raised 2,3DPG and raised temperature all cause the curve to shift to the right. Alkalosis, myoglobin and fetal Hb cause shift to the left. The shift caused by pH is called the Bohr effect

pressures of oxygen in blood is described by the oxygen-dissociation curve (Figure 2.3). It is sigmoid shaped because oxygen molecules demonstrate "positive cooperativity" when associating with Hb. Each Hb molecule carries four oxygen molecules. The first oxygen molecule helps the others to associate as well. The reason this curve is so important and clever is that large amounts of oxygen can be released from the blood for only a small drop in partial pressure in the capillaries (because of the steep lower part of the curve). Other local factors affect the curve, or the affinity of Hb to carry oxygen, like acidosis, which shifts it to the right. This means more oxygen is released in acidotic tissue, which needs it. The oxygen-dissociation curve flattens after 94% saturation (usually equivalent to a PaO_2 of 8·3 kPa or 64 mmHg).

Pulse oximetry

Cyanosis can be difficult to detect and one objective measurement of oxygenation is pulse oximetry. Oximetry measures the percentage saturation of haemoglobin and this indirectly relates to PaO_2 through the oxygen dissociation curve. This indirect relationship can lead to errors in clinical practice if one forgets that pulse oximetry measures saturation, not PaO_2. Red and infrared light are transmitted through the tissues by a light-emitting diode. A photodetector picks up the transmitted light and the ratio of light emitted to light absorbed is translated into a percentage saturation value. Inaccurate pulse oximeter readings arise from:

- light interference
- motion artefact
- low perfusion states
- abnormal haemoglobin.

Why PaCO2 rises

There is much misunderstanding around the causes of a high $PaCO_2$ in relation to oxygen therapy. For the purposes of explanation, "CO_2 retention" is the name used for the phenomenon that occurs because of uncontrolled oxygen therapy in patients with chronic hypoxaemia. "Hypercapnic respiratory failure" is the term used when the $PaCO_2$ rises for other reasons.

CO₂ retention

At one time it was thought that suppression of hypoxic drive was the cause of CO_2 retention. Changes in CO_2 is one of the main controls of ventilation in normal people. In patients with a chronically high CO_2 the chemoreceptors in the brain become blunted and the patient depends on hypoxaemia to stimulate ventilation, something that normally occurs only at altitude or during illness. If these patients are given too much oxygen, their "hypoxic drive" is abolished, breathing will slow, and $PaCO_2$ will rise as a result, causing CO_2 narcosis and eventually apnoea. Although this is the traditional explanation for CO_2 retention, some studies have shown that minute volume and respiratory rate are unchanged in such patients and alternative explanations are as follows:

- There is release of hypoxic vasoconstriction with oxygen therapy, with a change in ventilation–perfusion in the lung and an increase in dead space ventilation. Hypoxic vasoconstriction is an important physiological mechanism in normal people, designed to improve the match between perfusion and ventilation by diverting blood away from poorly ventilated areas. Patients with COPD have a poor chemical drive for breathing and compensatory hyperventilation does not occur.
- There is a reduced ventilatory drive in some patients with COPD, both in response to hypercapnia and hypoxaemia. The reasons for this are not really known, but genetic factors play a part (the "normal" family members of hypercapnic COPD patients often demonstrate blunted hypercapnic and hypoxaemic responses). Acquired loss of drive as an adaptation to increased work of breathing is also implicated. In "CO_2 retainers" a different pattern of ventilation has been observed, with lower tidal volumes but an increased respiratory rate. This could be a compensatory mechanism designed to reduce the work of breathing.
- The *Haldane effect* may also play a part. When haemoglobin is saturated with oxygen, the amount of carbon dioxide it can carry is reduced. Most CO_2 is carried in solution and when the affinity of haemoglobin for H^+ ions is reduced, the number of H^+ ions in solution increases as a result. Patients with COPD do not compensate.

Patients with severe mechanical impairment of lung function are susceptible to CO_2 retention as described above. This includes some, but by no means all, patients with COPD. Various studies show that when CO_2 retention exists, it occurs when the FEV1 is < 1·0 litre. It may be that these patients are particularly prone to CO_2 retention during an acute exacerbation of their illness. Other patients are also vulnerable to CO_2 retention for example those with obstructive sleep apnoea. Such patients require controlled oxygen therapy using a Venturi mask to get the PaO_2 to around 8·0 kPa (60 mmHg).

One in five patients with COPD admitted to hospital has a respiratory acidosis. The more severe the respiratory acidosis, the greater the mortality. Some of this acidosis is caused by uncontrolled oxygen therapy. A recent study looked at oxygen administration in 101 consecutive admissions via the Emergency Department in patients with COPD. The British Thoracic Society recommends that patients with COPD should receive 28% oxygen via a Venturi mask until the results of arterial blood gases are known. In this study 56% patients received more than 28% oxygen and the median time from ambulance to arterial blood gas analysis was 1 hour. In-hospital mortality was 14% for patients who received more than 28% oxygen and 2% for those who received 28% oxygen or less. Many patients identified their condition as asthma to the ambulance crew. This study was heavily criticised by subsequent letters which illustrate the ongoing debate on the cause of CO_2 retention and the correct use of oxygen therapy in acute exacerbations of COPD.

It is important to note that depriving a critically ill patient from oxygen can be harmful. Experts in critical care point out that hypoxaemia can be fatal. In certain circumstances it may be necessary to administer higher concentrations of oxygen to patients with COPD if they are acutely and severely hypoxaemic, pending ventilation.

Acute hypercapnic respiratory failure

Unfortunately, teaching on CO_2 retention as described above has been misunderstood so that many doctors persist in reducing the oxygen concentration in any patient who has a high $PaCO_2$. This is illogical and can be harmful. The most common reason for a high $PaCO_2$ is a problem with ventilation. This occurs when the load on the respiratory muscles is too great or there is respiratory muscle weakness (Figure 2.4).

Excessive load results from increased resistance (for example, upper or lower airway obstruction), reduced compliance (for example, infection, oedema, rib fractures, or obesity), and increased respiratory rate. Respiratory muscle weakness can be caused by a problem in any part of the neurorespiratory pathway starting in the brain and working down (for example, drug overdose, motor neurone disease, Guillain–Barré syndrome, myasthenia gravis, and electrolyte abnormalities – low potassium, magnesium, phosphate or calcium).

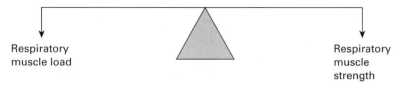

Respiratory
muscle load

Respiratory
muscle
strength

Figure 2.4 Hypercapnic respiratory failure and the balance between load and muscle strength

Hypercapnia as a result of ventilatory failure is important to recognise. Reducing the oxygen concentration in order to "treat" a high CO_2 is entirely the wrong thing to do in this situation. High concentrations of oxygen do not depress ventilation in patients with a high CO_2 caused by an imbalance between respiratory muscle load and strength. Correct treatment is of the underlying cause and assistance with ventilation.

Does my patient have chronic hypoxaemia/hypercapnia?

There are clues to help you decide whether or not your patient may be prone to CO_2 retention:

- Patients with chronic hypoxaemia develop compensatory responses – polycythaemia and pulmonary hypertension (or cor pulmonale). Look for these.
- Background history – what is the patient normally like and what medication is being taken? Are there any previous lung function tests?
- History of the acute episode.
- Analysis of admission arterial blood gases.

If your patient is young and normally fit and well you can be virtually certain that any rise in CO_2 is due to a problem with ventilation and nothing to do with oxygen therapy. If the acute diagnosis is a drug overdose, head injury, neuromuscular weakness, or acute left ventricular failure, the high CO_2 is due to a problem with ventilation. Note that patients with a background of COPD can also present with these problems. In terms of the history, a newly diagnosed patient with COPD who still goes hill-walking is less likely than a housebound patient on long-term oxygen therapy to have chronic hypoxaemia/hypercapnia. Analysis of the admission arterial blood gases can also give useful information. Both these patients have COPD:

- pH 7·36, $PaCO_2$ 9·0 kPa (65·3 mmHg), bicarbonate 35 mmol/l, BE +6, PaO_2 6·0 kPa (46 mmHg)
- pH 7·25, $PaCO_2$ 8·0 kPa (65·3 mmHg), bicarbonate 26 mmol/l, BE −2, PaO_2 8·0 kPa (62 mmHg)

The first is from a patient who has a chronically high $PaCO_2$ (because the pH is normal and the base excess is high). The hypoxaemia is also likely to be chronic. The second is from an acutely decompensated patient who is hypoxaemic and hypoperfused (because the base excess is low). This patient needs oxygen, assistance with ventilation and intravenous fluids. Non-invasive ventilation in COPD should be instituted early – as soon as the pH falls below 7·35 according to trials – because the further the degree of respiratory acidosis, the less the chances of recovery (see Chapter 4). Worsening respiratory acidosis may require intubation.

In summary:

- The most common cause of hypercapnia is a problem with ventilation – this has nothing to do with oxygen therapy.
- In patients with COPD, use Venturi masks titrated to arterial blood gases and institute non-invasive ventilation early where indicated.

Self-assessment – case histories

1. A 60-year-old lady arrives in the Emergency Department with breathlessness. She was given 12 litres per minute oxygen via a simple face mask by the paramedics. She is on inhalers for COPD, is a smoker, and a diabetic. She is clammy and has

widespread crackles and wheeze in the lungs. The chest x ray film has an appearance consistent with severe left ventricular failure. Her blood gases show: pH 7·15, $PaCO_2$ 8·0 kPa (61·5 mmHg), PaO_2 9·0 kPa (69·2 mmHg), bicarbonate 20 mmol/l, BE – 6. The attending doctor has taken the oxygen mask off because of "CO_2 retention" by the time you arrive. The oxygen saturations were 95% and are now 85%. Blood pressure is 140/70 mmHg. Comment on her oxygen therapy.

2. A 50-year-old man arrives in the Medical Admissions Unit with breathlessness. He is an ex-miner, has COPD, and is on inhalers at home. His blood gases on 28% oxygen show: pH 7·4, $PaCO_2$ 8·5 kPa (65·3 mmHg), PaO_2 8·5 kPa (65·3 mmHg), bicarbonate 38·4 mmol litre^{-1}, BE + 7. A colleague asks you if he needs non-invasive ventilation because of his hypercapnia. What is your reply?

3. A 30-year-old patient on the chemotherapy ward becomes unwell with breathlessness. The nurses report oxygen saturations of 75%. When you go to the patient, you find the other observations are as follows: pulse 130 per minute, blood pressure 70/40 mmHg, respiratory rate 40 per minute, patient confused. Blood gases on air show: pH 7·1, $PaCO_2$ 3·0 kPa (23 mmHg), PaO_2 11 kPa (115 mmHg), bicarbonate 6·8 mmol/l, BE – 20. The chest is clear. A chest x ray film is taken and is normal. Can you explain the oxygen saturations and the breathlessness?

4. A 50-year-old man is undergoing a urological procedure. As part of this, intravenous methylene blue is given. Shortly afterwards, the junior anaesthetist notices the patient's oxygen saturations drop suddenly to 70%. All the equipment seems to be working normally. Worried that the patient has had some kind of embolism, he calls his senior. What is the explanation?

5. A 45-year-old man arrives unconscious in the Emergency Department. There is no history available apart from the fact that he was found collapsed in his car by passers-by. On examination he is unresponsive, pulse 90 per minute, blood pressure 130/60 mmHg, oxygen saturations 98% on 15 litres per minute oxygen via a reservoir bag mask. His ECG shows widespread ST depression and his arterial blood gases show: pH 7·25, $PaCO_2$ 6·0 kPa (46 mmHg), PaO_2 7·5 kPa (57·6 mmHg), bicarbonate 19·4 mmol/l, BE – 10. His full blood count is normal. What is the explanation for the discrepancy in the SaO_2 and PaO_2?

6. A 25-year-old man with no past medical history was found on the floor at home having taken a mixed overdose of benzodiazepines and tricyclic antidepressant tablets. He is drowsy (Glasgow Coma Score is 8) and he has probably aspirated, because there is right upper lobe consolidation on the chest x ray film. He arrives hypothermic (34°C) and arterial blood gases on 15 litres per minute via a reservoir bag mask show: pH 7·2, $PaCO_2$ 9·.5 kPa (73 mmHg), PaO_2

12·0 kPa (92·3 mmHg), bicarbonate 27·3 mmol/l, BE +2. His blood pressure is 80/50 mmHg and his pulse is 120 per minute. The attending doctor changes his oxygen to a 28% Venturi mask because of his high CO_2 and repeat blood gases show: pH 7·2, $PaCO_2$ 9·0 kPa (69·2 mmHg), PaO_2 6·0 kPa (46·1 mmHg), bicarbonate 26 mmol/l, BE +1. What would your management be?

Self-assessment – discussion

1. This patient has COPD, but:

   - the problem is severe acute left ventricular failure (LVF);
   - acute hypoxaemia will aggravate cardiac ischaemia;
   - other aspects of the history and examination may give clues as to whether or not she is likely to have severe COPD.

   The arterial blood gases show a mixed respiratory and metabolic acidosis with relative hypoxaemia. Ventilatory failure owing to LVF is the main reason for the high $PaCO_2$ and needs treatment as soon as possible. Initial treatment should concentrate on A, B, C. Medical treatment for left ventricular failure is required. Intubation is indicated if there is no improvement. Non-invasive continuous positive airway pressure (CPAP) may be tried first in an ICU setting. The patient should not be hypoxaemic.

2. No. His pH is normal. His $PaCO_2$ is normally high (he has a high standard bicarbonate and BE to have fully compensated for his chronic respiratory acidosis). He should stay on a Venturi mask whilst unwell.

3. The main reason why this patient's oxygen saturations are so low is hypoperfusion. The PaO_2 is normal on air – this makes pulmonary embolism (PE) unlikely in someone so unwell (cancer and chemotherapy are two independent risk factors for PE). This patient has circulatory shock as illustrated by the low blood pressure and severe metabolic acidosis seen on the arterial blood gases. Shocked patients breathe faster because of circulatory hypoxia and metabolic acidosis. The history and examination will tell you whether or not this shock is due to bleeding (Are the platelets very low?) or severe sepsis (Is the white cell count very low?). Patients with septic shock do not always have the classical warm peripheries and bounding pulses – they can be peripherally vasoconstricted. Treatment priorities are A, B (including high concentration oxygen therapy), and C – the patient needs fluid. Oxygen delivery can be optimised by correcting any fluid deficit and improving cardiac output. Severe anaemia may require blood transfusion.

4. Methylene blue in the circulation affects oxygen saturation measurement. The apparently low saturations return to normal

within a few minutes. The junior anaesthetist did the right thing: he checked the airway (tube position), breathing (listened to the chest and checked the ventilator settings), and circulation (measured blood pressure and pulse) before asking for advice.

5. The arterial blood gases show a metabolic acidosis with hypoxaemia. The $PaCO_2$ is at the upper limit of normal. It should be low in a metabolic acidosis, indicating a relative respiratory acidosis as well. Treatment priorities in this patient are as follows: securing the airway and administering the highest concentration of oxygen possible, assessing and treating breathing problems, and correcting any circulation problems. There is a discrepancy between the SaO_2 of 98% and the arterial blood gas result, which shows a PaO_2 of 7·5 kPa (57·6 mmHg). Tied in with the history and ischaemic-looking ECG, the explanation for this is carbon monoxide (CO) poisoning. CO poisoning produces carboxyhaemoglobin seen by the pulse oximeter as oxyhaemoglobin causing an overestimation of saturations. CO poisoning is the commonest cause of death by poisoning in the UK. Mortality is especially high in those with pre-existing atherosclerosis. Toxicity is not just due to COHb formation. Free radicals, platelet activating factors and cytochrome AA3 formation also play a part. Loss of CO from the body is a slow process at normal atmospheric pressure and oxygen concentration (21%). It takes 4·5 hours for the concentration of CO to fall to half its original value (Table 2.2). CO removal is increased by increasing the oxygen concentration or by placing the victim in a hyperbaric chamber. This increases the amount of oxygen in the blood, forcing off CO.

Table 2.2 Half life of CO depending on conditions

Oxygen concentration	Half life of CO (minutes)
Room air (21%)	240–300
15 litres/min reservoir bag mask (80%)	80–100
Intubated and ventilated (with 100% oxygen)	50–70
Hyperbaric chamber (100% oxygen at 3 atmospheres)	20–25

There is debate as to whether treatment with hyperbaric oxygen is superior to ventilation with 100% oxygen on intensive care. Five randomised trials to date disagree. Therefore a pragmatic approach is recommended:

- any history of unconsciousness
- COHb levels of > 40% at any time

- neurological or psychiatric features at the time of examination
- pregnancy (because the fetal COHb curve is shifted to the left of the mother's)
- ECG changes

are all features that lead to hyperbaric oxygen being considered – but the risks of transporting critically ill patients to a hyperbaric unit also needs to be taken into account. Ventilation with 100% oxygen is an acceptable alternative, and treatment with high concentrations of oxygen should continue for a minimum of 12 hours.

6. This is a 25-year-old man with no previous medical problems. He does not have chronic hypoxaemia. He will not "retain CO_2" – he has a problem with ventilation. The arterial blood gases show an acute respiratory acidosis with a lower PaO_2 than expected. He has a reduced conscious level so his airway needs to be secured. He needs a high concentration of oxygen (that is, 15 litres per minute via a reservoir bag mask) until he is intubated. He has several reasons to have a problem with ventilation – reduced conscious level, aspiration pneumonia, and respiratory depressant drugs. With regards to circulation, he needs volume expansion with warmed fluids. The combination of cardiac toxins he has taken with superimposed hypoxaemia and hypoperfusion could lead to cardiac arrest. Sodium bicarbonate infusion is indicated in severe tricyclic poisoning (see Chapter 9). Flumazenil (a benzodiazepine antidote) is not advised when significant amounts of tricyclic antidepressants have also been taken as it reduces the fit threshold. It is worth measuring creatinine kinase levels in this case as rhabdomyolysis (from lying on the floor for a long time) will affect fluid management.

Further reading

Baldwin DR and Allen MB. Non-invasive ventilation for acute exacerbations of chronic obstructive pulmonary disease. *BMJ* 1997;**314**:163–4.

British Thoracic Society. Guidelines for the management of acute exacerbations of COPD. *Thorax* 1997;**52**(Suppl 5):S16–21.

Calverley PMA. Oxygen-induced hypercapnia revisited. *Lancet* 2000;**356**: 1538–39.

Davies RJO and Hopkin, JM. Nasal oxygen in exacerbations of ventilatory failure: an underappreciated risk. *BMJ* 1989;**299**:43–4.

Denniston AKO, O'Brien C, Stableforth D. The use of oxygen in acute exacerbations of COPD: a prospective audit of pre-hospital and hospital emergency management. *Clin Med* 2002;**2**:449–51.

Robinson TD, Freiberg DB, Regnis JA, Young IH. The role of hypoventilation and ventilation-perfusion redistribution in oxygen-induced hypercapnia during acute exacerbations of COPD. *Am J Respir Crit Care Med* 2000;161:1524–9

Various authors. The use of oxygen in acute exacerbations of COPD: a prospective audit of pre-hospital and hospital emergency management [letters]. *Clin Med* 2003;3:183–6.

3: Acid-base balance

By the end of this chapter you will be able to:

- understand how the body maintains a narrow pH
- know the common causes of acid-base abnormalities
- understand why the arterial blood gas is one of the first investigations in any critically ill patient
- interpret arterial blood gas reports and calculate the anion gap
- apply this to your clinical practice

Acid as a by-product of metabolism

The human body continually produces acid as a by-product of metabolism. However, it must also maintain a stable pH, which is necessary for normal enzyme activity and the millions of chemical reactions that take place in the body each day. Normal blood pH is 7·35–7·45. This is maintained by:

- intracellular buffers, for example proteins and phosphate
- then by extracellular buffers, for example plasma proteins, haemoglobin and carbonic acid/bicarbonate
- finally the kidneys and lungs.

A buffer is a substance that resists pH change by absorbing or releasing hydrogen ions (H^+) when acid or base is added to it. The carbonic acid/bicarbonate system is the most important buffer – more effective at buffering acid than base. The relationship between CO_2, carbonic acid and bicarbonate is quite clever:

$$H_2O + CO_2 \leftrightarrow H_2CO_3 \leftrightarrow HCO_3^- + H^+$$
Carbonic anhydrase

Unlike other buffer systems, the components of the carbonic acid/bicarbonate system can be varied independently of one another. Adjusting the rate of alveolar ventilation changes CO_2 levels and the kidneys regulate H^+ excretion in the urine. The excretory functions of the lungs and kidneys are connected by H_2CO_3 (carbonic acid). This ensures that if one organ becomes overwhelmed, the other can help or "compensate".

The lungs have a simple way of regulating CO_2 excretion, but the kidneys have three main ways of excreting H^+:

- by regulating the amount of HCO_3^- absorbed (80–90% is reabsorbed in the proximal tubule);
- by the reaction: $HPO_4^{2-} + H^+ \rightarrow H_2PO_4^-$. The H^+ comes from carbonic acid, leaving HCO_3^-, which passes into the blood;
- by combining ammonia with H^+ from carbonic acid. The resulting ammonium ions cannot pass back into the cells and are excreted.

The kidney produces HCO_3^- which reacts with free hydrogen ions. This results in a fall in serum HCO_3^- concentration, which is why in a metabolic acidosis, the serum HCO_3^- is low.

pH and the Henderson–Hasselbach equation

H^+ ions are difficult to measure as there are literally billions of them. We use pH instead, which simply put is the negative logarithm of the H^+ concentration in moles.

$$pH = -\log [H^+]$$

Buffers are weak acids. When a weak acid dissociates:

$$AH \leftrightarrow A^- + H^+$$

where A is the acid and AH is the conjugate base, the product of [A] and [H^+] divided by [AH] remains constant. Put in equation form:

$$Ka = \frac{[A^-] \cdot [H^+]}{[AH]}$$

Ka is called the dissociation constant. pKa is like pH – it is the negative logarithm of Ka. The Henderson–Hasselbach equation puts the pH and the dissociation equations together and describes the relationship between pH and the molal concentrations of the dissociated and undissociated form of a dissolved substance.

The Henderson–Hasselbach equation is:

$$pH = pK + \log \frac{[\text{conjugate base}]}{[\text{acid}]}$$

A simplified version is:

$$pH \propto \frac{[HCO_3^-] \text{ dissociated}}{PaCO_2 \text{ undissociated}}$$

H + concentration is sometimes used instead of pH. A simple conversion between pH 7·2 and 7·5 is that [H+] = 80 – the two digits after the decimal point. So if the pH is 7·35, [H+] is 80 – 35 = 45 nmol/l.

From the law of mass action:

$$[H+] = Ka \times \frac{PaCO_2}{HCO_3}$$

or

$$[H+] = \frac{181 \times PaCO_2 \text{ in kPa } (24 \times PaCO_2 \text{ in mmHg})}{HCO_3}$$

[H+] is related to the $PaCO_2/HCO_3$ ratio. This is clinically relevant when checking the consistency of arterial blood gas data.

Table 3.1 pH and equivalent [H+]

pH	[H+] nmol/l
7·6	26
7·5	32
7·4	40
7·3	50
7·2	63
7·1	80
7·0	100
6·9	125
6·8	160

Compensation versus correction

Normal acid-base balance is a normal pH (euphaemia) plus a normal $PaCO_2$ and HCO_3. Compensation is normal pH even though the HCO_3^- and $PaCo_2$ are disturbed. Correction is the restoration of normal pH, HCO_3^- and $PaCO_2$ through correction of the underlying cause. Acidaemia is a low pH whereas acidosis is a high $PaCO_2$ or a low bicarbonate. In the same way, alkalaemia is a high pH whereas alkalosis is a low $PaCO_2$ or high bicarbonate. Acidosis and alkalosis refer to *processes* that tend to lower or raise pH. Compensatory mechanisms rarely restore the pH to normal. Thus a normal pH in the presence of an abnormal HCO_3^- and $PaCO_2$ immediately suggests a mixed disorder.

The base excess and standard bicarbonate

The base excess and base deficit measure how much extra acid or base is in the system as a result of a metabolic problem. The base excess is calculated by measuring the amount of strong acid that has to be added to the sample to produce a normal pH of 7·4 – it is therefore taking into account all the buffer systems. Minus is a base deficit (that is, the sample is already acidotic so no acid has to be added). Plus is a base excess (that is, the sample is alkalotic so acid has to be added). The normal range is – 2 to + 2 mmol/l. Base deficit can be an important predictor of severity of illness (see Chapter 5).

Standard bicarbonate is the concentration of bicarbonate in a sample kept under standard conditions – 37°C with a $PaCO_2$ of 5·3 kPa (40 mmHg). This is calculated from the actual bicarbonate. Standard bicarbonate therefore purely reflects the metabolic component of acid-base balance as opposed to any subsequent changes in bicarbonate occurring as a result of respiratory problems.

Common causes of acid-base disturbances

Changes in pH occur because of:

- abnormal respiratory function
- abnormal renal function
- an overwhelming acid or base load.

Table 3.2 Changes in pH, $PaCO_2$ and bicarbonate in different acid-base disturbances

	pH	$PaCO_2$	base excess	standard bicarbonate
Respiratory acidosis	low	high	normal	normal
Metabolic acidosis	low	normal	low	low
Respiratory alkalosis	high	low	normal	normal
Metabolic alkalosis	high	normal	high	high

Since [H+] is regulated by two systems – the respiratory system and the kidneys – there are four possible primary acid-base disorders:

- respiratory acidosis (acute or chronic)
- metabolic acidosis (further divided into increased or normal anion gap)
- respiratory alkalosis (acute or chronic)
- metabolic alkalosis (further divided into saline responsive and saline unresponsive).

A summary of the changes in pH, $PaCO_2$ and bicarbonate in the different acid-base disturbances is shown in Table 3.2.

Respiratory acidosis

Respiratory acidosis is caused by alveolar hypoventilation. Alveolar hypoventilation is not the same as a reduced respiratory rate – a person may be breathing at a normal or high rate but have a reduced minute volume (= frequency × tidal volume). Acute alveolar hypoventilation results from an imbalance between respiratory muscle strength and load (see previous chapter). Chronic alveolar hypoventilation as seen in chronic obstructive pulmonary disease (COPD) involves multiple mechanisms.

In acute respiratory acidosis, compensation occurs firstly by cellular buffering over minutes to hours. Renal compensation then occurs over 3–5 days.

Metabolic acidosis

Metabolic acidosis usually arises from an increased acid load but can also be due to loss of bicarbonate. Respiratory compensation occurs within minutes. Maximal compensation occurs within 12–24 hours, but respiratory compensation is limited by the work involved in breathing and the systemic effects of a low carbon dioxide. It is unusual for the body to be able to fully compensate for a metabolic acidosis.

The anion gap

Blood tests measure most cations (positively charged molecules) but only a few anions (negatively charged molecules). Anions and cations are equal in the human body, but if we add all the measured cations and anions together there will be a gap – this reflects the concentration of those anions not measured, for example plasma proteins, phosphates, and organic acids. This is called the anion gap and is calculated by:

$$(Na + K) - (chloride + HCO_3)$$

The normal range is 10–16 mmol litre^{-1}. In an increased anion gap metabolic acidosis, the body has gained an acid load. In a normal anion gap metabolic acidosis, the body has usually lost bicarbonate. Causes of an increased anion gap metabolic acidosis include (Box 3.1):

- excess acid through ingestion
- excess acid through the body's own production
- excess acid through an inability to excrete.

In a normal anion gap metabolic acidosis, bicarbonate is lost via the gastrointestinal tract (diarrhoea or ileostomy) or the kidneys (tubular damage or acetazolamide therapy). Occasionally there is reduced renal H$^+$ excretion.

Change in anion gap versus change in HCO$_3$

If there is an increased anion gap, it may be helpful to relate this to the fall in plasma HCO$_3$. Fifty per cent of excess H+ is buffered by cells and not by HCO$_3$, but most of the excess anions remain in the extracelluar fluid as they cannot cross the cell membrane. Therefore, the increase in anion gap

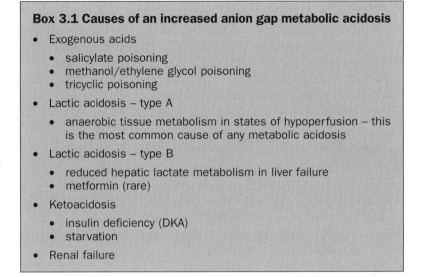

Box 3.1 Causes of an increased anion gap metabolic acidosis

- Exogenous acids
  - salicylate poisoning
  - methanol/ethylene glycol poisoning
  - tricyclic poisoning
- Lactic acidosis – type A
  - anaerobic tissue metabolism in states of hypoperfusion – this is the most common cause of any metabolic acidosis
- Lactic acidosis – type B
  - reduced hepatic lactate metabolism in liver failure
  - metformin (rare)
- Ketoacidosis
  - insulin deficiency (DKA)
  - starvation
- Renal failure

usually exceeds the fall in plasma HCO_3. In lactic acidosis the ratio is around 1·6 to 1·0. In ketoacidosis the ratio is nearer 1·0 to 1·0 because of the loss of ketoacids in the urine which does not occur in lactic acidosis. Thus, calculating the change in anion gap versus change in HCO_3 can help differentiate ketoacidosis from other acidosis.

Mini-tutorial: the use of intravenous sodium bicarbonate in metabolic acidosis

HCO_3^- as sodium bicarbonate may be administered intravenously to raise blood pH in severe metabolic acidosis but this has several problems. It increases the formation of CO_2, which passes readily into cells (unlike HCO_3^-). This worsens intracellular acidosis. Some compromised patients may need ventilation to counter the increased CO_2 production caused by an infusion of sodium bicarbonate. The oxygen-dissociation curve is shifted to the left by alkalosis leading to impaired oxygen delivery to the tissues. Sodium bicarbonate contains a significant sodium load and because 8·4% solution is hypertonic, the increase in plasma osmolality can lead to vasodilatation and hypotension. Tissue necrosis can result from extravasation from the cannula. Many of the causes of metabolic acidosis respond to restoration of intravascular volume, tissue perfusion, and treatment of the underlying cause. For these reasons, intravenous sodium bicarbonate is not often used in metabolic acidosis; 8·4% sodium bicarbonate = 1 mmol ml^{-1} of sodium or bicarbonate.

Respiratory alkalosis

Respiratory alkalosis is caused by alveolar hyperventilation – the opposite of respiratory acidosis. The kidneys take 2–5 days to compensate fully by excreting bicarbonate in the urine and retaining hydrogen ions. Many people tend to think that "hyperventilation" means hysteria. This is incorrect. Hyperventilation is a sign, not a diagnosis, and it has many causes:

- shock
- lung causes (hypoxaemia, pulmonary embolism, pneumonia, pneumothorax, pulmonary oedema)
- CNS causes (meningitis/encephalitis, raised intracranial pressure, stroke, cerebral haemorrhage)
- metabolic causes (fever, acute liver failure, hyperthyroidism)
- drugs (salicylate poisoning)
- Gram-negative septicaemia
- psychogenic causes (pain, anxiety).

Metabolic alkalosis

Metabolic alkalosis is the least well known of the acid-base disturbances. It can be divided into two groups: saline responsive and saline unresponsive. Saline responsive metabolic alkalosis is the most common and occurs with volume contraction, for example diuretic use or volume depletion. Urinary chloride is low in the saline responsive type. Vomiting or nasogastric suction leads to loss of hydrochloric acid, but the decline in glomerular filtration rate that accompanies this perpetuates the metabolic alkalosis. The kidneys try to reabsorb chloride (hence the urine levels are low), but there is less of it from loss of hydrochloric acid, so the only available anion to be reabsorbed is bicarbonate. Metabolic alkalosis is often associated with hypokalaemia, owing to secondary hyperaldosteronism from volume depletion.

Another cause of saline responsive metabolic alkalosis is when hypercapnia is quickly corrected. Post-hypercapnia alkalosis occurs because hypercapnia directly affects the proximal tubules and decreases sodium chloride reabsorption

Table 3.3 Changes in pH, $PaCO_2$, base excess and standard bicarbonate in different acid-base disturbances.

Acid-base disturbance	pH	$PaCO_2$	Base excess	Standard bicarbonate
Respiratory acidosis	Low	High	Normal	Normal
Metabolic acidosis	Low	Normal	Low	Low
Respiratory alkalosis	High	Low	Normal	Normal
Metabolic alkalosis	High	Normal	High	High

leading to volume depletion. If chronic hypercapnia is corrected rapidly with mechanical ventilation, metabolic alkalosis ensues because there is already a high bicarbonate and the kidney needs time to excrete it. The pH change causes hypokalaemia, which can lead to cardiac arrhythmias.

Saline unresponsive metabolic alkalosis occurs due to renal problems:

- with high blood pressure – excess mineralocorticoid (exogenous or endogenous)
- with normal blood pressure – severe low potassium, high calcium
- exogenous alkali with low glomerular filtration rate

A summary of the changes in pH, $PaCO_2$, and base excess in different acid-base disturbances is shown in Table 3.3.

Interpreting an arterial blood gas report

Arterial blood gas analysis can be performed quickly and gives useful information about A (oxygenation), B (ventilation) and C (perfusion) – which is why it is one of the first tests (with bedside glucose measurement) performed in critical illness. However, many clinicians fail to carry out a full analysis and benefit from information that could influence therapy.

The box below describes the 6 steps in arterial blood gas analysis:

1. Is the data consistent?
2. What is the primary acid-base abnormality? An abnormal pH always indicates the primary acid-base disturbance – the body never overcompensates
3. Check the appropriateness of compensation – there may be more than one acid-base disturbance
4. Measure the anion gap in any metabolic acidosis
5. Look at PaO_2 – the A-a gradient may reveal disorders of oxygenation (see chapter 4)
6. Finally, consider the clinical situation – does the analysis fit with the clinical picture?

For example, in the following arterial blood gas: pH 7·25, $PaCO_2$ 4·5 kPa (35 mmHg) bicarbonate 14·8 mmol/l, PaO_2 8·0 kPa (61 mmHg), there is a metabolic acidosis. pH 7·25 = [H+] 55 nmol/l. From the law of mass action we can see that the data is consistent – that is, there is no lab error.

$$[H+] = \frac{181 \times 4·5 \text{ in kPa}}{14·8} = 55$$

Metabolic acidosis is the primary diagnosis. But although the $PaCO_2$ is "normal" in this example, it is possible to estimate what the $PaCO_2$ should be from compensatory responses empirically derived from human studies (see Table 3.4).

In this example there should be a 0·15 kPa (1·2 mmHg) fall in $PaCO_2$ for every 1 mmol/l fall in HCO_3. Assuming the lower limit of normal for HCO_3 is 22 mmol/l, there has been a 7 mmol/l fall in HCO_3 which should cause a 1·1 kPa (8·4 mmHg) fall in $PaCO_2$. The $PaCO_2$ in this example should be 3·4 kPa. It is "normal" because there is also a respiratory acidosis. This alerts you to the fact that the patient may be sicker than at first thought. Mixed acid-base disorders are common in clinical practice.

Normal arterial blood values are: pH 7·35–7·45, $PaCO_2$ 4·5–6·0 (35–46 mmHg), PaO_2 11–14·5 kPa (83–108 mmHg), BE –2 to +2, bicarbonate 22–28 mmol/l. Useful information on acid-base balance can easily be gained from venous blood; oxygenation, however, cannot be interpreted.

Table 3.4 Compensatory responses

Disorder	Primary change	Compensatory response
Metabolic acidosis	Reduction in HCO_3	0·15 kPa (1·2 mmHg) fall in $PaCO_2$ for every 1 mmol/l fall in HCO_3
Metabolic alkalosis	Increase in HCO_3	0·01 kPa (0·7 mmHg) increase in $PaCO_2$ for every 1 mmol/l rise in HCO_3
Acute respiratory acidosis	Increase in $PaCO_2$	1 mmol/l increase in HCO_3 for every 1·3 kPa (10 mmHg) rise in $PaCO_2$
Chronic respiratory acidosis	Increase in $PaCO_2$	3·5 mmol/l increase in HCO_3 for every 1·3 kPa (10 mmHg) rise in $PaCO_2$
Acute respiratory alkalosis	Reduction in $PaCO_2$	2·0 mmol/l reduction in HCO_3 for every 1·3 kPa (10 mmHg) fall in $PaCO_2$
Chronic respiratory alkalosis	Reduction in $PaCO_2$	5·0 mmol/l reduction in HCO_3 for every 1·3 kPa (10 mmHg) fall in $PaCO_2$

Self-assessment – case histories

1. A 65-year-old man with COPD comes to the Emergency Department with shortness of breath. His arterial blood gases on air show: pH 7·29, $PaCO_2$ 8·5 (65·3 mmHg), standard bicarbonate 30·5 mmol/l, BE +4, PaO_2 8·0 kPa (62 mmHg). What is the acid-base disturbance and what is your management?

2. A 60-year-old ex-miner with COPD is admitted with shortness of breath. His arterial blood gases on air show: pH 7·36, $PaCO_2$ 9·0 (65·3 mmHg), standard bicarbonate 35 mmol/l, BE +6, PaO_2 6·0 (46·1 mmHg). What is the acid-base disturbance and what is your management?

3. A 24-year-old man with epilepsy comes to hospital in status epilepticus. He is given intravenous diazepam. Arterial blood gases on 10 l/min oxygen via reservoir bag mask show: pH 7·05, $PaCO_2$ 8·0 (61·5 mmHg), standard bicarbonate 16 mmol/l,

BE −8, PaO_2 15 kPa (115 mmHg). His other results are sodium 140 mmol/l, potassium 4·0 mmol/l and chloride 98 mmol/l. What is his acid-base status and why?

4. A patient is admitted in a coma from a drug overdose and responds only to painful stimuli. Arterial blood gases on air show: pH 7·24, $PaCO_2$ 8·32 (64 mmHg), standard bicarbonate 29 mmol/l, BE +2, PaO_2 7·8 kPa (60 mmHg). The Emergency Department doctor diagnoses drug intoxication with aspiration pneumonia because of the hypoxaemia. What is your assessment?

5. Twenty-four hours later you are asked to assess the same patient for discharge. She has woken up and the arterial blood gases have improved: pH 7·60, $PaCO_2$ 3·1 (24 mmHg), standard bicarbonate 22 mmol/l, BE −2, PaO_2 9·1 kPa (70 mmHg). The hospital is in need of beds. Should you discharge this patient?

6. An 80-year-old lady is admitted with abdominal pain. Her vital signs are normal, apart from cold peripheries and a tachycardia. Her arterial blood gases on air show: pH 7·1, $PaCO_2$ 3·5 (30 mmHg), PaO_2 9·5 kPa (73 mmHg), standard bicarbonate 8 mmol/l, BE −15. You review the clinical situation again – she has generalised tenderness in the abdomen but it is soft. Her blood glucose is 6·0 mmol/l (100 mg/dl), sodium 140 mmol/l, potassium 3·7 mmol/l, chloride 89 mmol/l, urea 6·5 mmol/l (BUN 18 mg/dl). There are reduced bowel sounds. The chest x ray is normal. The ECG shows atrial fibrillation. What is the reason for the acid-base disturbance?

7. A 44-year-old man comes to the Emergency Department with pleuritic chest pain and shortness of breath which he has had for five days. A moderately sized pneumothorax is seen on the chest x ray. His arterial blood gases on 10 l/min oxygen via simple face mask show: pH 7·44, $PaCO_2$ 3·0 (23 mmHg), standard bicarbonate 16·0 mmol/l, BE −4, PaO_2 30·5 (234·6 mmHg). Is there a problem with acid-base balance?

8. A patient is admitted to hospital with breathlessness and arterial blood gases on air show: pH 7·2, $PaCO_2$ 4·1 (31·5 mmHg), standard bicarbonate 36 mmol/l, BE +10, PaO_2 7·8 (60 mmHg). Can you explain this?

9. A 45-year-old woman with a history of peptic ulcer disease reports six days of persistent vomiting. On examination she has a blood pressure of 100/60 mmHg and looks dehydrated. Her blood results are as follows: sodium 140 mmol/l, potassium 2.2 mmol/l, chloride 86 mmol/l, bicarbonate 40 mmol/l, urea 29 mmol/l (BUN 80 mg/dl), pH 7·5, $PaCO_2$ 6·2 kPa (53 mmHg), PaO_2 14 (107 mmHg), urine pH 5·0, urine sodium 2 mmol/l, urine potassium 21 mmol/l and urine chloride 3 mmol/l. What is the acid-base disturbance? How would you treat this patient? Twenty-four hours after appropriate therapy the HCO_3 level is 30 mmol/l. The following urine values are obtained: pH 7·8, sodium 100 mmol/l, potassium 20 mmol/l and chloride

3 mmol/l. How do you account for the high urine sodium but low chloride concentration?

10. A 50-year-old alcoholic is brought in to the Emergency Department unconscious. He had appeared drunk beforehand with ataxia and slurred speech and has slowly lapsed into a coma. On examination he is unresponsive and has nystagmus. His vital signs are: respiratory rate 30/min, blood pressure 190/100 mmHg, pulse 110/min, temperature 36OC. His bedside glucose measurement is 5 mmol/l (83 mg/dl). His arterial blood gases on 10 litres oxygen via reservoir bag mask show: pH 7·15, $PaCO_2$ 3·0 (23 mmHg), standard bicarbonate 7·6 mmol/l, BE −20, PaO_2 40 (308 mmHg). His full blood count, liver enzymes and clotting are normal. Other results are: sodium 145 mmol/l, potassium 5 mmol/l, urea 3 mmol/l, creatinine 100 µmol/l, chloride 80 mmol/l. What do these arterial blood gases show? What is the cause of his unconsciousness?

11. Match the clinical history with the appropriate arterial blood gas values:

	pH	$PaCO_2$	HCO_3 (mmol/l)
a	7·39	8·45 kPa (65 mmHg)	37
b	7·27	7·8 kPa (60 mmHg)	26
c	7·35	7·8 kPa (60 mmHg)	32

- A severely obese 24-year-old man
- A 56-year-old woman with COPD who is started on diuretic therapy for peripheral oedema resulting in 3 kg weight loss
- A 14-year-old girl with a severe asthma attack

12. A 50-year-old man is recovering on the surgical ward ten days after a total colectomy for bowel obstruction. He has type 1 diabetes and is on an intravenous insulin sliding scale and his ileostomy is working normally. His vital signs are: BP 150/70, respiratory rate 16/min, SaO_2 98% on air, urine output 1500 ml/day, temperature normal and he is alert. Abdominal examination is normal and he is well perfused. The surgical team are concerned about his persistently high potassium level (which was noted before surgery) and metabolic acidosis. His blood results are: sodium 130 mmol/l, potassium 6·5 mmol/l, urea 14 mmol/l (BUN 39 mg/dl), creatinine 180 µmol/l (2·16 mg/dl), chloride 109 mmol/l, 8am cortisol 500 nmol/l (18 µg/dl). He is known to have diabetic nephropathy and is on Ramipril. His arterial blood gases on air show: pH 7·29, $PaCO_2$ 3·5 kPa (27 mmHg), PaO_2 14 kPa (108 mmHg), bicarbonate 12 mmol/l. What is his acid-base disturbance and why? Should the surgeons request a CT scan of the abdomen to look for a cause for his acidosis?

Self-assessment – discussion

1. Is the data consistent? Yes – [H+] = 181 × 8·5/30·5 = 50 nmol/l which is pH 7·3. There is an acidaemia (low pH) with a high $PaCO_2$ – a primary respiratory acidosis. The fact that the pH is abnormal indicates an acute change (or "decompensation"). There should be a 1 mmol/l increase in HCO_3 for every 1·3 kPa (10 mmHg) rise in $PaCO_2$ in an acute respiratory acidosis. The $PaCO_2$ has risen by 2·5 kPa above the upper limit of normal so HCO_3 should rise by around 2 mmol/l – as in this case. Management starts with assessment/treatment of the airway, breathing and circulation, followed by a quick assessment of disability (neurology), bedside glucose measurement, arterial blood gases, further information gathering and definitive treatment. Non-invasive ventilation is appropriate in this case if simple measures fail to improve the respiratory acidosis quickly.

2. Is the data consistent? Yes – [H+] = 181 × 9·0/35 = 46·5 nmol/l which is pH 7·36. There is a normal pH (euphaemia) despite a high $PaCO_2$ (respiratory acidosis). This is due to compensation. There should be a 3·5 mmol/l increase in HCO_3 for every 1·3 kPa (10 mmHg) rise in $PaCO_2$. The $PaCO_2$ has risen by 3·0 kPa above the upper limit of normal, so HCO_3 should rise by around 8 mmol/l. The measured HCO_3 is consistent at 35 mmol/l. Management includes assessment/treatment of airway, breathing, circulation and disability (neurology). A 28% Venturi mask is appropriate oxygen therapy, titrated to arterial PaO_2 and $PaCO_2$ plus treatment for his exacerbation of COPD.

3. Is the data consistent? Yes – [H+] = 181 × 8·0/16 = 90·5 nmol/l which is pH 7·05. There is both a raised $PaCO_2$ and a reduced HCO_3 suggesting mixed respiratory and metabolic acidosis. The anion gap is 26 mmol/l which is raised. The change in anion gap is 10 (upper limit of normal is 16) versus a change in HCO_3 of 6 (lower limit of normal is 22). This ratio is raised and is suggestive of lactic acidosis. This interpretation is consistent with the clinical scenario – the patient has a lactic acidosis from fitting and a respiratory acidosis due to intravenous diazepam. This acid-base disturbance should spontaneously return to normal with supportive measures.

4. Is the data consistent? Yes – [H+] = 181 × 8·32/27 = 56 nmol/l which is pH 7·24. There is an acidaemia with a raised $PaCO_2$ – the primary disturbance is a respiratory acidosis. In acute respiratory acidosis there should be a 1 mmol/l increase in HCO_3 for every 1·3 kPa (10 mmHg) rise in $PaCO_2$. The $PaCO_2$ has risen by 2·3 kPa above the upper limit of normal so HCO_3 should be around 29 mmol/l, which it is. The anion gap cannot be measured in this case without further information. The A-a gradient (see chapter 4) is normal in this case – suggesting that the hypoxaemia is due to alveolar hypoventilation rather than pneumonia.

5. Is the data consistent? Yes – [H+] = 181 × 3·1/22 = 26 nmol/l which is pH 7·6. There is alkalaemia with a low $PaCO_2$ – a primary respiratory alkalosis. The fall in $PaCO_2$ from 4·5 kPa (lower limit of normal) to 3·1 kPa should result in a reduction in HCO_3 by nearly 4 mmol/l. The measured bicarbonate of 22 mmol/l is consistent. The A-a gradient (see chapter 4) is now raised which indicates that the respiratory alkalosis is due to intrinsic lung disease, for example, aspiration pneumonia. This analysis fits with the clinical picture. The patient should not be discharged.

6. Is the data consistent? Yes – [H+] = 181 × 3·5/8 = 80 nmol/l which is pH 7·1. There is acidaemia with a low HCO_3 and low $PaCO_2$ – a primary metabolic acidosis. There should be a 0·15 kPa (1·2 mmHg) fall in $PaCO_2$ for every 1 mmol/l fall in HCO_3. HCO_3 has fallen from 22 (the lower limit of normal) to 8 mmol/l so $PaCO_2$ should fall by 14 × 0·15 which is 2·1 kPa. The $PaCO_2$ should be 2·4 kPa. The measured $PaCO_2$ of 3·5 kPa indicates an accompanying respiratory acidosis. The anion gap is (140 + 3·7) – (89 + 8) = 46·7 mmol/l which is high. The change in anion gap versus the change in bicarbonate is 30·7/14 and this suggests lactic acidosis. The A-a gradient is slightly elevated which could indicate developing SIRS (see chapter 7). Is this analysis in keeping with the clinical picture? Yes – the combination of abdominal pain and a lactic acidosis should alert you to the possibility of intra-abdominal ischaemia. The elderly show few signs of an inflammatory response because of their less active immune system. The presence of atrial fibrillation is a clue to this diagnosis. Priorities in the management of this case are: assessment and treatment of the airway, breathing, circulation and disability followed by analgesia, further information gathering and definitive treatment.

7. Is the data consistent? Yes – [H+] = 181 × 3·0/15·1 = 36 nmol/l which is pH 7·44. Although the pH is normal, acid-base status is not. How can we tell which acid-base disturbance occurred first – the low $PaCO_2$ or the low bicarbonate? By considering the clinical picture. Given the history of breathlessness for a few days, we can say the low $PaCO_2$ due to hyperventilation occurred first. This is a compensated respiratory alkalosis. In a chronic respiratory alkalosis, there should be a 5·0 mmol/l reduction in HCO_3 for every 1·3 kPa (10 mmHg) fall in $PaCO_2$. The $PaCO_2$ has fallen by 1·5 kPa below the lower limit of normal so the HCO_3 should have fallen by just over 5·0 mmol/l – which it has in this case. Increased minute ventilation in normal pregnancy also causes a compensated respiratory alkalosis. This can cause confusion if the patient is being investigated for possible pulmonary embolism. The A-a gradient is not affected.

8. Is the data consistent? No – [H+] = 181 × 4·1/36 = 20 nmol/l which is pH 7·7. As you may have guessed, this is an impossible blood gas – the answer is lab error!

9. Is the data consistent? Yes − $[H+] = 181 \times 6\cdot9/40 = 31$ nmol/l which is pH 7·5. The results show an alkalaemia with a raised HCO_3 and $PaCO_2$ is a primary metabolic alkalosis. There should be a 0·01 kPa (0·7 mmHg) increase in $PaCO_2$ for every 1 mmol/l rise in HCO_3. The HCO_3 has risen by 12 mmol/l above the upper limit of normal so $PaCO_2$ should rise by $12 \times 0\cdot01 = 0\cdot12$ kPa. The expected $PaCO_2$ is 6·12 kPa which is roughly the measured level. The physical findings and low urinary sodium levels point to volume depletion. The patient should be treated with both intravenous sodium chloride and potassium chloride. During therapy, volume expansion reduces sodium reabsorption in order to correct the metabolic alkalosis by excreting excess HCO_3. The discrepancy between urinary sodium and chloride is primarily due to urinary HCO_3 excretion. Urinary $PaCO_2$ is similar to renal venous $PaCO_2$ so from the law of mass action:
Urinary $[H+]$ 16 nmol/l = $181 \times 6\cdot2$/urinary bicarbonate
Urinary bicarbonate may be calculated as 70 mmol/l
Further chloride replacement is necessary for as long as chloride depletion exists. Low urinary chloride may be seen as a marker of continuing volume depletion.

10. Is the data consistent? Yes − $[H+] = 181 \times 3\cdot0/7\cdot6 = 72$ nmol/l which is pH 7·15. These results show a primary metabolic acidosis. There should be a 0·15 kPa (1·2 mmHg) fall in $PaCO_2$ for every 1 mmol/l fall in HCO_3. The HCO_3 has fallen by 14·4 so $PaCO_2$ should fall by $14\cdot4 \times 0\cdot15$ or 2·16 kPa. The expected $PaCO_2$ level is 2·3 kPa. There is an accompanying respiratory acidosis, probably due to fatigue. The anion gap is $(145 + 5) − (80 + 5) = 65$ mmol/l which is very large. Poisoning, lactic/keto acidosis or renal failure are candidates. In this case poisoning is the most likely cause, given the normal liver tests, glucose and creatinine levels. Certain poisons characteristically cause a huge anion gap and are more commonly ingested by alcoholics − ethylene glycol (antifreeze) and methanol. These can be measured in the serum to confirm the diagnosis. Alternatively, the osmolal gap can be calculated. This is the difference between the calculated and actual osmolality of the serum. The calculated osmolality is as follows:

$$\frac{1\cdot86 \times \text{sodium} + \text{urea} + \text{glucose}}{0\cdot93}$$

In normal individuals the osmolal gap is less than 10 mosmol/kg H2O. In ethylene glycol poisoning it is raised, reflecting the unmeasured presence of ethylene glycol in the serum. Specific treatment consists of alcohol dehydrogenase inhibitors − either alcohol or 4-methylpyrazole (4-MP). Intravenous ethanol (alcohol) therapy requires frequent monitoring of blood alcohol levels, aiming for 100–150 mg/dl.

4-MP is more expensive but easier to administer, does not cause central nervous system depression and has more predictable pharmacokinetics. Management in this case is to secure the airway and give oxygen, assist ventilation and assess/treat circulatory abnormalities before moving on to a full examination, information gathering and definitive treatment.

11. From the history:

- Severe obesity suggests chronic hypercapnia (c)
- COPD and diuretic therapy suggests chronic hypercapnia with superimposed metabolic alkalosis (a)
- A severe asthma attack suggests acute respiratory acidosis (b)

12. Is the data consistent? Yes – $[H+] = 181 \times 3 \cdot 5/14 = 53$ nmol/l which is pH 7·29. The results show a primary metabolic acidosis. The expected $PaCO_2$ is 3·1 kPa. The anion gap is $(130 + 6 \cdot 5) - (14 + 109) = 13 \cdot 5$ mmol/l which is normal. The PaO_2 is normal on air. In a normal anion gap metabolic acidosis, bicarbonate is lost via the gastrointestinal tract (diarrhoea, fistula or uterosigmoidostomy) or the kidneys (tubular damage or acetazolamide therapy). Sometimes there is reduced renal H+ excretion. In this case there are no excess gastrointestinal losses, leaving the possibility of a renal problem, which fits with the clinical setting of diabetic nephropathy. Renal tubular acidosis is a collection of disorders where the kidneys either cannot excrete H+ or generate HCO_3^-. Serum potassium can help differentiate the types (see Table 3.5).

Table 3.5 Renal tubular acidosis

	Problem	GFR	Serum potassium
Type 1 (distal)	Distal H+ secretion	Normal	Low
Type 2 (proximal)	Proximal H+ secretion	Normal	Low
Type 3 (glomerular insufficiency)	NH_3 production (hence HCO_3 generation)	Reduced	Normal
Type 4 (hyporeninaemic hypoaldosteronism	Distal sodium reabsorption, potassium secretion and H+ secretion	Reduced	High

GFR = glomerular filtration rate

Hyporeninacmic hypoaldosteronism is commonly found in diabetic nephropathy and hypertensive renal disease. ACE inhibitors, spironolactone and NSAIDs (which further reduce aldosterone levels) worsen the hyperkalaemia. Treatment consists of restricting dietary potassium and using fludrocortisone or bicarbonate supplements. Based on these findings and the clinical examination the surgeons do not need to request a CT scan of the abdomen.

Further reading

Burton David Rose, Theodore Post. *Clinical physiology of acid-base disorders* (5th edition). New York: McGraw-Hill, 2000.
Driscoll P, Brown T, Gwinnutt C, Wardle T. *A simple guide to blood gas analysis.* London: BMJ Publishing Group, 1997.

4: Respiratory failure

By the end of this chapter you will be able to:

- classify respiratory failure according to arterial blood gases
- know about the alveolar gas equation
- understand about different types of ventilatory support
- apply this to your clinical practice

Definitions

The major function of the respiratory system is to supply the blood with adequate oxygen and to remove carbon dioxide. This process is achieved by three distinct mechanisms:

- ventilation – the delivery and removal of air to and from the alveoli
- diffusion – oxygen and carbon dioxide cross the alveolar-capillary wall
- circulation – transported from the site of gas exchange to the cells and back again.

To accomplish this, the lungs function as an area of gas exchange and as a pump for effective ventilation. Failure of these two functions results in hypoxaemia or hypercapnia respectively. Hence respiratory failure is traditionally defined as hypoxaemic respiratory failure (PaO_2 < 8·0 kPA or 60 mmHg) or hypercapnic respiratory failure (hypoxaemia with $PaCO_2$ above 6·0 kPA or 50 mmHg).

Respiratory failure may be classified as three main types:

- hypoxaemia – mainly an imbalance between ventilation and perfusion in the lung
- hypercapnia – an imbalance between ventilatory capacity and demand
- a mixture of hypoxaemia and hypercapnia, commonly seen in clinical practice.

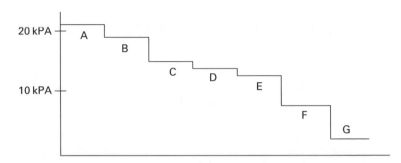

Figure 4.1 Oxygen partial pressure (vertical lines) in parts of the body (horizontal lines). A, inspired dry gas; B, humidified at 37°C; C, mixed with expired gas; D, alveolar ventilation and O_2 consumption; E, venous mixing and $\dot{V}/\dot{Q}$ mismatch; F, capillary blood concentration depends on blood flow and haemoglobin concentration; G, mitochondria

Hypoxaemia

Cardiac output is important in the delivery of oxygen to the tissues. The proportion of oxygen delivery increased by increasing the PaO_2 or SaO_2 when it is already above the shoulder of the haemoglobin–oxygen dissociation curve is small compared with improving a reduced cardiac output. Therefore in the management of the critically ill patient as much attention should be paid to fluid resuscitation as to the normalisation of hypoxaemia (see Chapter 2).

Oxygen tension in the air is around 20 kPA (154 mmHg) at sea level, falling to 0·5 kPA (3·8 mmHg) in the mitochondria. This gradient is known as the oxygen "cascade" (Figure 4.1). An interruption at any point can cause hypoxia – high altitude, upper or lower airway obstruction, alveolar flooding, abnormal haemoglobins, circulatory failure and mitochondrial poisoning are examples.

Hypoxaemic respiratory failure is characterised by a low PaO_2, leading to an elevated alveolar–arterial oxygen gradient and a low $PaCO_2$, reflecting adequate ventilation but inadequate gas exchange. Hypoxaemia is most commonly due to the mismatch of ventilation ($\dot{V}$) and perfusion ($\dot{Q}$) or intrapulmonary right-to-left shunts (Figure 4.2).

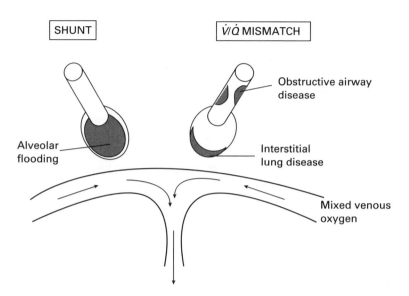

Figure 4.2 Ventilation/perfusion mismatch and shunts

$\dot{V}/\dot{Q}$ mismatch

If an airway supplying a region of the lung is impaired by the presence of secretions or narrowed by bronchoconstriction, that segment will be perfused but only partially ventilated. The resulting $\dot{V}/\dot{Q}$ mismatch will result in hypoxaemia, but giving supplemental oxygen will cause the PaO_2 to increase.

Intrapulmonary right-to-left shunts

If an alveolus is totally filled with fluid or collapsed, the segment will be perfused but not ventilated at all. Mixed venous blood is shunted across that segment. Increasing the inspired oxygen in the presence of a moderate to severe shunt will not improve PaO_2. Intrapulmonary shunting as a cause of hypoxaemia is observed in pneumonia and atelectasis.

$\dot{V}/\dot{Q}$ mismatch and intrapulmonary shunting can often be distinguished by the response of the patient to supplemental oxygen.

The A–a gradient

The A–a gradient is a measure of the drop in partial pressure of oxygen between the alveolus and arterial blood. It can be estimated from the arterial blood gases. A PaO_2 of 14 kPA (107 mmHg) could be considered normal – until one realises that the patient is breathing 60% oxygen. The predicted PaO_2 should be approximately 8 kPA (75 mmHg) below the FiO_2. There is a significant problem with gas exchange in this example. This problem can be measured by the A–a gradient. In some situations, the A–a gradient can be a more sensitive measure than PaO_2 alone in indicating a problem with gas exchange.

Alveolar oxygen can be estimated using the alveolar gas equation. Oxygen leaves the alveolus in exchange for carbon dioxide. The amount of CO_2 entering the alveolus is known as this is almost the same as arterial CO_2. Slightly less CO_2 is excreted than O_2 absorbed so a correction factor (0·8) is added.

The alveolar gas equation is:

$$PAO_2 = PiO_2 \ (PB - PAH_2O) - PACO_2/0·8$$

where PB equals the ambient barometric pressure which equals 101 kPA at sea level and PAH_2O equals the alveolar partial pressure of water which equals 6 kPA. This is often simplified to:

$$PAO_2 = PiO_2 - PACO_2/0·8$$

Once PAO_2 has been estimated, the A–a gradient ($PAO_2 - PaO_2$) can be calculated. Any significant difference is due to abnormal gas exchange. Normal people have a small difference because the bronchial veins of the lung and thebesian veins of the heart carry unsaturated blood to the left ventricle, bypassing the alveoli. A normal A–a gradient is up to 2 kPA (15 mmHg) or 4 kPA (30 mmHg) in smokers and the elderly.

A person breathing air with a PaO_2 of 12·0 kPA and a $PaCO_2$ of 5·0 kPA has an A–a gradient as follows:

$$0·21 \times 95 - 5/0·8$$

When calculating the A–a gradient on air, 0.21×95 is often shortened to 20:

$$20 - 5/0.8 = 13.75$$

The A–a gradient is:

$$13.75 - 12 = 1.75 \text{ kPA}$$

The calculation of the A–a gradient illustrates the importance of always documenting the inspired oxygen concentration. Relative hypoxaemia cannot be detected without this.

Hypercapnia

The reasons why $PaCO_2$ rises are often misunderstood. This is explained in detail in Chapter 2. To summarise:

- "CO_2 retention" is the phenomenon that occurs with uncontrolled oxygen therapy in patients with chronic hypoxaemia (for example, some patients with COPD).
- Hypercapnic respiratory failure – or ventilatory failure – has nothing to do with oxygen therapy. Ventilatory capacity is the amount of spontaneous ventilation that can be maintained without the development of respiratory muscle fatigue. Normally ventilatory capacity matches demand. Hypercapnic respiratory failure results from either a reduction in ventilatory capacity or an increase in ventilatory demand – or both.

Metabolism rapidly generates acid. The metabolism of fats and carbohydrates leads to the formation of a large amount of CO_2. This combines with water to form carbonic acid. The lungs excrete the volatile fraction through ventilation. Ventilation is influenced and regulated by chemoreceptors for $PaCO_2$, PaO_2, and pH located in the brainstem as well as by neural impulses from lung stretch receptors and impulses from the cerebral cortex. $PaCO_2$ is determined by the balance between CO_2 production and its removal via alveolar ventilation. This can be expressed by the equation:

$$PaCO_2 \propto \dot{V}co_2/\dot{V}A$$

where $\dot{V}co_2$ is the rate of delivery of CO_2 to the alveoli by capillary blood and $\dot{V}a$ is the rate of removal of CO_2 by alveolar ventilation.

CO_2 production is increased in hypermetabolic states and by infusions of sodium bicarbonate. At a constant rate of carbon dioxide production, $PaCO_2$ is determined by the level of alveolar ventilation. A decrease in alveolar ventilation can result either from reduced minute ventilation or increased dead space.

Mixed hypoxaemic and hypercapnic respiratory failure

The functions of the lung as a pump and as an area of gas exchange are not independent. Disease commonly causes problems with both. A good example of this is seen postoperatively. Surgery causes atelectasis because of a combination of supine position, general anaesthesia, and pain. A reduction in functional residual capacity below closing volume also contributes to hypoxaemia. Good analgesia, chest physiotherapy, and early mobilisation help to prevent this. Excessive load from reduced compliance and increased minute volume in combination with opiates which depress respiration lead to hypercapnia. At risk patients are those with pre-existing lung disease, who are obese, or who have upper abdominal or thoracic surgery.

Treatments for respiratory failure

Any patient with acute respiratory failure should be admitted to a respiratory care unit or other level 2–3 facility. Hypoxaemia is the most life-threatening facet of respiratory failure. The goal is to ensure adequate oxygen delivery to tissues which is generally achieved with a PaO_2 above 8·0 kPA (60 mmHg) or SaO_2 of at least 94%. However, patients who normally have hypoxaemia, hypercapnia, and breathlessness require different therapeutic targets than patients without lung disease. One would not necessarily aim for "normal" values in such patients.

Apart from oxygen therapy (see Chapter 2), various types of respiratory support are used to treat respiratory failure. These can be extremely confusing for the uninitiated. A simplified

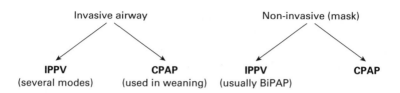

Figure 4.3 Different types of respiratory support. Modes of IPPV (intermittent positive pressure ventilation): volume control; pressure control; pressure support; synchronised intermittent mandatory ventilation; biphasic positive airway pressure (BiPAP)

version is as follows. As well as treatment of the underlying cause (for example, antibiotics for pneumonia), the lungs can be supported in the following ways:

- through an invasive airway, for example the patient is intubated
- non-invasive respiratory support via a tight-fitting mask.

Whether the patient is intubated or has a tight-fitting mask, various modes of respiratory support exist (Figure 4.3), which are described below.

The most important decision when faced with a person with acute respiratory failure is to decide which should be the first line method of respiratory support. Some situations require intubation whereas others can be managed non-invasively.

Non-invasive ventilation (NIV) is contraindicated in:

- patients with recent facial or upper airway surgery, facial burns or trauma
- vomiting
- recent upper gastrointestinal surgery, bowel obstruction
- inability to protect own airway
- copious respiratory secretions
- other organ system failure, for example haemodynamic instability
- severe confusion/agitation.

Table 4.1 First-line methods of respiratory support in different conditions

Intubation	Non-invasive ventilation (NIV or BiPAP)	Non-invasive CPAP
Asthma	COPD pH 7·25—7·35	Acute cardiogenic pulmonary oedema
ARDS	Decompensated sleep apnoea	Hypoxaemia in chest trauma
Severe respiratory acidosis	Acute on chronic hypercapnic respiratory failure due to chest wall deformity/ neuromuscular disease	
Any cause with impaired conscious level		
Pneumonia*		

*If NIV or CPAP is used as a trial of treatment in pneumonia or postoperative respiratory failure, this should be done on an ICU with close monitoring and rapid access to intubation. ARDS, acute respiratory distress syndrome; BiPAP, bilevel positive airway pressure; COPD, chronic obstructive pulmonary disease; CPAP, continuous positive airway pressure; NIV, non-invasive ventilation.

However, NIV is sometimes used in drowsy or confused patients if it is decided that the patient is not suitable for intubation because of severe chronic lung disease.

The effects of ventilation

Spontaneous ventilation can be assisted or replaced by delivering an intermittent positive pressure to the lungs. This is what happens when an unconscious patient is ventilated by hand with a bag and mask. In the past "iron lungs" were used to apply an intermittent negative pressure to the thorax, but manual intermittent positive pressure ventilation (IPPV) was introduced during a large polio epidemic in Copenhagen in 1952. Mortality rates were much more favourable than those following previously used techniques. This heralded the introduction of intensive care units.

During IPPV there is reversal of the thoracic pump – the normal negative intrathoracic pressure during spontaneous inspiration, which draws blood into the chest from the vena cavae, a significant aspect of venous return. With IPPV, venous return decreases during inspiration and, if a positive pressure is added during expiration as well (positive end-expiratory pressure or PEEP), venous return will be impeded throughout the respiratory cycle. This can cause hypotension. The degree of impairment of venous return is directly proportional to the mean intrathoracic pressure. So changes in ventilatory pattern, not just pressures, can cause cardiovascular changes.

At high lung volumes the heart may be directly compressed by lung expansion. This prevents adequate filling of the cardiac chambers. Ventricular contractility is also affected. Elevated intrathoracic pressures directly reduce the left and right ventricular ejection pressure which is the difference between the pressure inside and outside the ventricular wall during systole. As a result, stroke volume is reduced for a given end-diastolic volume. This is usually detrimental, but in failing hearts IPPV can improve cardiac output by reducing filling pressures and returning the heart to a more favourable portion on the Frank–Starling curve.

IPPV indirectly produces an overall decline in renal function with a reduced urine volume and sodium excretion. Hepatic function can also be adversely affected by the decrease in cardiac output, with increased vascular resistance and elevated bile duct pressure. The gastric mucosa does not have an autoregulatory capability. Therefore mucosal ischaemia and surgical bleeding may result from a decreased cardiac output and an increased gastric venous pressure.

These physiological changes during IPPV can be precipitously revealed when intubating critically ill patients. Marked hypotension and cardiovascular collapse can occur as a result of uncorrected volume depletion prior to intubation. This is compounded by the administration of anaesthetic drugs, which vasodilate and reduce circulating catecholamine levels as patients lose consciousness.

The effects on cardiac output are seen in both invasive and non-invasive IPPV, but the effects are not as dramatic in non-invasive ventilation as the patient is awake and breathing spontaneously, with the ventilator acting only as an assistant.

Table 4.2 Advantages and disadvantages of volume versus pressure control

Parameters	Volume control	Pressure control
Delivery	Delivers a set tidal volume no matter what pressure this requires. This can cause barotrauma	If airway pressures are high, only small tidal volumes will be delivered. Not good if lung compliance keeps changing
Leaks	Poor compensation	Compensates for leaks well (e.g. poor fitting mask or circuit fault)
PEEP	Many volume control ventilators cannot apply PEEP	PEEP easily added

PEEP, positive end-expiratory pressure.

Specific modes of IPPV

Ventilators that deliver IPPV are set to deliver either a certain volume or a certain pressure. This is termed "volume-control" or "pressure-control" ventilation and the different characteristics have advantages and disadvantages (Figure 4.2).

In volume-controlled ventilation, inhalation proceeds until a preset tidal volume is delivered and this is followed by passive exhalation. A feature of this mode is that gas is delivered at a constant inspiratory flow, resulting in peak pressures applied to the airways higher than that required for lung distension. Since the volume delivered is constant, airway pressures vary with changing pulmonary compliance and airway resistance. A major disadvantage is that excessive airway pressure may be generated, resulting in barotrauma.

In pressure-control ventilation a peak inspiratory pressure is applied and the pressure difference between the ventilator and lung results in inflation until that pressure is attained. Passive exhalation follows. The delivered volume is dependent on pulmonary and thoracic compliance. A major advantage of pressure control is the decelerating inspiratory flow pattern, in which inspiratory flow tapers off as the lung inflates. This usually results in a more homogeneous gas distribution throughout the lungs. A major disadvantage is that dynamic changes in pulmonary mechanics may result in varying tidal volumes.

More sophisticated ventilators have been manufactured, mainly for intensive care units, which incorporate the characteristics of both modes (for example, pressure-limited volume control). Alarms have been added for excessive leaks and abnormally high or low pressures and volumes. Some examples are illustrated below:

- Pressure support ventilation (PSV) – PSV is patient-initiated, pressure-control ventilation. The ventilator assists in response to the patient's spontaneous inspiratory effort. With each inspiratory effort the ventilator delivers a preset pressure.
- Synchronised intermittent mandatory ventilation (SIMV) – the ventilator delivers preset breaths (for example, 12 per minute) in coordination with the respiratory effort of the patient. Spontaneous breathing is allowed between breaths. Synchronisation attempts to limit barotrauma, which can occur if a preset breath is delivered to a patient who is already in maximal inhalation or is forcefully exhaling.
- Biphasic or bilevel positive airway pressure (BiPAP) – this delivers a continuous positive airway pressure (CPAP) that cycles between a higher and a lower positive pressure.

The pressure waveforms of different ventilation modes are shown in Figure 4.4.

Additional ventilator settings typically include breaths per minute, inspired oxygen concentration, the ratio of inspiration to expiration, inspiratory and expiratory pressures, pressure limits, and tidal volume measurements. In this way the dual lung functions of oxygenation and ventilation can be manipulated.

Weaning from invasive ventilation

Weaning is the progressive reduction in respiratory support as respiratory failure improves. The respiratory muscles become deconditioned during prolonged ventilation so an abrupt withdrawal of ventilatory support is often unsuccessful. Weaning is appropriate when the underlying

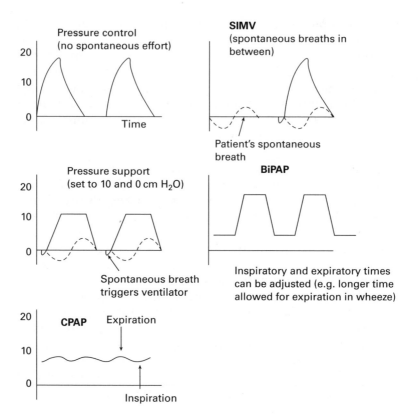

Figure 4.4 Pressure waveforms of different ventilation modes (cm H_2O)

cause of respiratory failure has been treated, other organ systems are stable, an appropriately low level of FiO_2 is required and PEEP is 5 cm H_2O or less. Some ventilatory modes are better than others during the weaning process, although limited evidence exists. There is usually a reduction in pressure support and a trial of breathing unsupported before extubation occurs. The rapid shallow breathing index has been studied extensively and is the best measurement to predict successful weaning. It measures the respiratory rate:tidal volume ratio during a 1-minute trial of breathing unsupported through a T-piece. Patients who develop more rapid and shallow breathing are unlikely to manage without ventilatory support. The cut-off figure is 105 – so a patient with 20 breaths per minute and tidal volumes of 0·5 litres has a rapid shallow breathing index of 40 and is likely to wean successfully, whereas a patient with 40 breaths per minute and tidal volumes of 0·25 litres has an index of 160 and is unlikely to manage unsupported.

Mini-tutorial: intubation in acute severe asthma

Intubation can be a life-saving intervention. Therefore it is important that it is performed early if indicated, particularly in acute severe asthma. A few minutes preparation beforehand is time well spent, particularly in those who are most unstable, as cardiovascular collapse can occur from uncorrected volume depletion, the abolition of catecholamine responses, and vasodilatation when general anaesthesia is given. Patients are volume loaded prior to intubation and a vasopressor (for example, ephedrine) is kept ready to treat hypotension. Anaesthetic drugs are given cautiously to minimise any vasodilatory effect and drugs that cause histamine release are avoided if possible. In life-threatening asthma, maximum medical therapy includes less commonly used bronchodilators, such as nebulised or subcutaneous adrenaline, intravenous salbutamol, magnesium sulphate, ketamine, and volatile anaesthetic agents. Once intubated, the patient is ventilated to allow a long expiratory time and this may mean only 6–8 breaths per minute is possible. "Permissive hypercapnia" is the term used when the $PaCO_2$ is allowed to rise in such situations, in order to prevent "stacking". In asthma, if the next positive pressure is delivered before there has been enough time for expiration to occur, the lung volume slowly expands, reducing venous return and leading to a progressive fall in cardiac output. The resulting hypotension which occurs is corrected by disconnecting the ventilator and allowing passive expiration to occur (which can take several seconds).

Non-invasive ventilation

Non-invasive ventilators are usually much simpler than those found on the ICU, with less settings to choose from. This is because most are designed for home use. The disadvantage of this is that they also tend to be poorly equipped in terms of monitoring and alarms when used in hospital. Home NIV will not be discussed here. The recent trials of NIV in exacerbations of COPD have used pressure-controlled ventilators. BiPAP (Respironics Inc.) is a commonly used pressure control ventilator in acute respiratory units in the UK.

Acute NIV should be considered in patients with mild to moderate acute respiratory failure (hypercapnia causing a pH of 7·2–7·35). The patient should have an intact airway, protective airway reflexes and be alert enough to follow commands. A common method is to begin with the expiratory level (EPAP) at 5 cm H_2O and the inspiratory level (IPAP) at 15 cm H_2O. The levels are adjusted based on patient comfort, tidal volume achieved (if measured), and arterial blood gases. The main indications for acute NIV are:

- exacerbation of COPD with a mild to moderate respiratory acidosis
- weaning from invasive ventilation.

The only condition for which there is conclusive evidence for acute NIV is acute exacerbations of COPD (see mini-tutorial below). NIV can also be used as a step-down treatment in patients who have been intubated and ventilated on ICU. Failure to wean exceeds 60% in COPD patients and this is a major cause of prolonged ICU stay and ICU costs. A recent randomised multicentre trial has shown that NIV is more successful in weaning than a conventional approach in patients with COPD. Patients who failed a T-piece trial (breathing spontaneously with no support) 48 hours after intubation were randomly assigned to receive either NIV immediately after extubation or conventional weaning (a gradual reduction in pressure support). The NIV group took a shorter time to wean, had shorter ICU stays, a lower incidence of hospital-acquired pneumonia, and increased 60-day survival. Other studies have reported similar findings.

Reports conflict regarding the efficacy of NIV in acute respiratory failure from other conditions such as ARDS and pneumonia. Earlier trials of NIV in pneumonia were discouraging, but a recent prospective randomised trial of NIV in community acquired pneumonia (56 patients) showed a significant fall in respiratory rate and the need for intubation. Just under one half of the patients in this study had COPD and it was carried out in an ICU with ready access to intubation. Generally, NIV failure rates are higher in non-COPD patients. NIV should never be used in acute severe asthma.

Mini-tutorial: NIV for exacerbations of COPD

An exacerbation of COPD requiring admission to hospital carries a 6–26% mortality. One study found a 5-year survival of 45% after discharge and this reduced to 28% with further admissions. Invasive ventilation in COPD carries a 50% or less survival to discharge. Ventilator-associated pneumonia is common and increases mortality still further. NIV is associated with less complications than intubation (Table 4.3).

Table 4.3 Complications of NIV versus intubation

NIV	Intubation
Necrosis of skin over bridge of nose	Pneumonia
Aspiration	Barotrauma and volutrauma
Changes in cardiac output (less)	changes in cardiac output
	complications of sedation
	and paralysis tracheal
	stenosis/tracheomalacia

Most studies of NIV in acute exacerbations of COPD have been performed in critical care areas. The majority used ICU ventilators with a face mask as opposed to custom-built NIV ventilators. The studies performed in general ward areas involved patients with a pH of > 7·29. There have been at least half a dozen prospective randomised controlled trials of NIV in acute exacerbations of COPD. The studies performed in ICUs showed a reduction in intubation rates and some also showed reduced mortality when compared with conventional medical therapy. None has directly compared NIV with intubation. A recent multicentre randomised controlled trial of NIV in general respiratory wards showed both a reduced need for intubation and reduced hospital mortality. Patients with a pH of < 7·3 after initial treatment did less well and it has been recommended that this group is managed in an ICU.

NIV should be commenced as soon as the pH falls below 7·35 because the further the degree of acidosis, the less the chances are of improvement. It should be used as an adjunct to full medical therapy, which treats the underlying cause of acute respiratory failure. However, in a 1-year prevalence study of 954 patients admitted with an exacerbation of COPD to one hospital, 25% were acidotic on arrival in the Emergency Department, but their pH was normal by the time they were admitted to a ward. This included patients with an initial pH of < 7·25, which suggests that NIV should be commenced after controlled oxygen and medical therapy has been administered.

Patients on NIV require close supervision because sudden deterioration can occur at any time. Simple measures such as adjusting the mask to reduce excessive air leaks can make a difference to the success or otherwise of treatment. Basic vital signs measured frequently give a indication of whether or not NIV is effective or failing. If NIV does not improve pH and respiratory rate in the first 2 hours, intubation should be considered. Predictors of failure of NIV in acute COPD are as follows:

- no improvement within 2 hours
- high APACHE II score (acute physiological and chronic health evaluation)
- pneumonia
- very underweight patient
- neurological compromise
- pH < 7·2 prior to starting NIV.

Non-invasive CPAP

Non-invasive CPAP was first introduced in the 1980s as a therapy for obstructive sleep apnoea (OSA). This is when a tight-fitting face or nasal mask delivers a single pressure throughout the patient's respiratory cycle. It is therefore not ventilation. In OSA, CPAP prevents pharyngeal collapse. CPAP can also be delivered through an endotracheal tube or tracheostomy tube in spontaneously breathing patients and is usually used this way during weaning. The application of a continuous pressure keeps the alveoli open for longer and improves oxygenation. This is therefore the main indication for CPAP.

The main indications for acute non-invasive CPAP are:

- to deliver increased oxygen in pneumonia or postoperative respiratory failure associated with atelectasis – this should be performed in an ICU;
- acute cardiogenic pulmonary oedema (see below).

CPAP is employed in patients with acute respiratory failure to correct hypoxaemia. In the spontaneously breathing patient, the application of CPAP provides positive end-expiratory pressure (PEEP) that can reverse or prevent atelectasis, improve functional residual capacity, and oxygenation. These improvements may prevent the need for

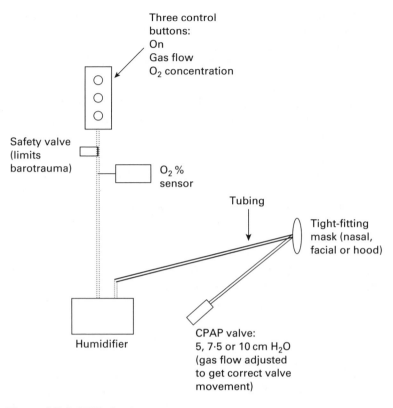

Figure 4.5 A CPAP circuit

endotracheal intubation. The inspiratory flow in a CPAP circuit needs to high enough to match the patient's peak inspiratory flow rate. If this is not achieved the patient will breathe against a closed valve with the risk that the generation of significant negative intrapleural pressure will lead to the development of pulmonary oedema. Always look at the expiratory valve in patients on CPAP. The valve should always remain slightly open during inspiration (Figure 4.5).

CPAP in patients with acute cardiogenic pulmonary oedema

One can think of acute cardiac failure in terms of "forward failure" (the inability to drive the circulation) or "backward failure" (the congestion caused by an inefficient pump). Backward failure causes pulmonary oedema and is often associated with a normal or high blood pressure. Treatment aims toward off-loading the heart. Medical therapy does this by

- sitting the patient up which reduces venous return, and
- giving frusemide, diamorphine and nitrates for their vasodilator properties.

When medical therapy fails, intubation may be the next step, but there are several studies that show that non-invasive CPAP reduces the need for intubation by reducing afterload and improving left ventricular function as well as its effects on the lungs.

Meta-analysis shows that non-invasive CPAP reduces the need for intubation in patients with acute cardiogenic pulmonary oedema (numbers needed to treat = 4) with a trend towards a reduction but no significant difference in mortality.

The respiratory effects of non-invasive CPAP are:

- Fluid is "squeezed" out of the alveoli into the circulation – there is a decline in the level of shunt because of redistribution of lung water from the alveolar space to the perivascular cuffs. PEEP reduces extravascular lung water and increases lymphatic flow through the thoracic duct in animal studies.
- PEEP prevents the collapse of alveoli at end-expiration, improving oxygenation.

The cardiac effects of non-invasive CPAP are:

- Left ventricular function is improved because afterload is reduced (leading to an increase in stroke volume). This occurs because the increased intrathoracic pressure has a squeezing effect on the left ventricle. There is a subsequent reduction in the pressure gradient between the ventricle and the aorta which has the effect of reducing the work required during contraction, that is, afterload.

- Relief of respiratory distress leads to haemodynamic improvement and reversal of hypertension and tachycardia – probably through reduced sympathoadrenergic stimulation.
- Sedation and a large reduction in venous return, which would be caused by high intrathoracic pressures, is avoided. These occur in intubated patients.

Non-invasive CPAP in acute cardiogenic pulmonary oedema is indicated when the patient has failed to respond to maximum medical therapy and there is an acute respiratory acidosis, unacceptable fatigue or hypoxaemia despite supplemental oxygen. Patients who do not respond quickly to CPAP should be considered for intubation.

Assessing the patient with respiratory failure

A, B, C, D, E is still the way to approach any patient, including one with respiratory failure (Box 4.1)

Box 4.1 Approach to a patient with respiratory failure

A
- relieve any upper airway obstruction
- administer oxygen

B
- count respiratory rate
- treat wheezing, fluid, consolidation or pneumothorax
- assess oxygen saturations and arterial blood gases
- consider if ventilatory support is required early and if so, what method

C
- fluid therapy
- treat any associated severe sepsis (see Chapter 7)

D
- assess conscious level as this affects treatment options

E
- full history and examination once A, B and C are stable

Self-assessment – case histories

1. A 30-year-old lady is admitted with acute severe asthma. Her vital signs are as follows: BP 100/60 mmHg, pulse 130, RR 40 per minute with poor respiratory effort, temperature 37°C and she is drowsy. Her arterial blood gases on 10 litres per minute reservoir bag mask show: pH 7·15, $PaCO_2$ 9·0 kPA (70 mmHg), PaO_2 7 kPA (54 mmHg), bicarbonate 22 mmol/l, BE − 5. What is your management?

2. Later on ICU the same patient develops hypotension (60/30 mmHg). The patient is paralysed and the ventilator is set to 12 breaths per minute. The inspiratory to expiratory ratio is 1:4, tidal volumes are 600 ml, and peak airway pressures are 45 cm H_2O. She is on volume-controlled ventilation. What are the possible causes of the hypotension and what is your management?

3. A 50-year-old man is admitted with an exacerbation of his COPD. His arterial blood gases on 28% oxygen (Venturi mask) show: pH 7·3, $PaCO_2$ 8·0 kPA (62 mmHg), PaO_2 7 kPA (54 mmHg) bicarbonate 29 mmol/l, BE + 3. What is your management?

4. A 40-year-old man with no past medical history is admitted with a severe pneumonia. His vital signs are: BP 120/70 mmHg, pulse 110, RR 40 per minute, temperature 38°C and he is alert. His arterial blood gases on 15 litres per minute via a reservoir bag mask show: pH 7·31, $PaCO_2$ 4·0 kPA (31·mmHg), PaO_2 6 kPA (46 mmHg), bicarbonate 14 mmol/l, BE − 8. What do you do?

5. You are called to see a 70-year-old man who is 2 days post-laparotomy. He has developed a cough with green phlegm and fever. His respiratory rate is increased (30 per minute) and his arterial blood gases on 10 litres per minute simple face mask show: pH 7·3, $PaCO_2$ 8·0 kPA (62 mmHg), PaO_2 7·6 kPA (58 mmHg), bicarbonate 29 mmol/l, BE + 4. What is your management?

6. A 60 kg 25-year-old lady with Guillain–Barré syndrome has been undergoing twice-daily forced vital capacity (FVC) measurements and treatment with intravenous immunoglobulin. Her FVC has fallen below 1 litre and her arterial blood gases on air now show: pH 7·3, $PaCO_2$ 7·5 kPA (58 mmHg), PaO_2 10 kPA (77 mmHg), bicarbonate 27 mmol/l, BE + 3. Her respiratory rate is 28 per minute. What do you do?

7. A 60-year-old man is admitted with acute severe left ventricular failure. He has been given 100 mg intravenous frusemide, salbutamol nebulisers, and a small dose of intravenous diamorphine. His arterial blood gases on 10 litres per minute oxygen via a reservoir bag mask show: pH 7·15, $PaCO_2$ 7 kPA (54 mmHg), PaO_2 9 kPA (70 mmHg), bicarbonate 18 mmol/l, BE − 8. His blood pressure is 180/90 mmHg and his respiratory rate is 38 per minute. What is your next step?

8. A 50-year-old lady is admitted with breathlessness. On examination she has an unrecordable blood pressure (which is 80 systolic by palpation). Her pulse is 110 per minute, RR 36 per minute, and she is alert. The chest sounds clear. The ECG shows sinus tachycardia with right heart strain and her chest x ray film

is normal. The arterial blood gases on 15 litres per minute via a reservoir bag mask show: pH 7·25, $PaCO_2$ 3·0 kPA (23 mmHg), PaO_2 12 kPA (92 mmHg), bicarbonate 10 mmol/l, BE – 12. What is the diagnosis and what is your management?

9. A 70-year-old man with COPD is admitted *in extremis*. He has been more breathless for a few days. He responds to painful stimuli only, his blood pressure is 130/60 mmHg, pulse 120 per minute and arterial blood gases on air show: pH 7·1, $PaCO_2$ 14·0 kPA (108 mmHg), PaO_2 6 kPA (46 mmHg), bicarbonate 20 mmol/l, BE – 4. What is your management?

10. A 30-year-old man arrives with pleurisy. There seems to be no obvious explanation for this and he has had a previous DVT. Calculate the A–a gradient using the arterial blood gas sample taken whilst the patient is breathing air. pH 7·5, $PaCO_2$ 4·0 kPa (30·7 mmHg) bicarbonate 24 mmol/l, BE 0, PaO_2 10·0 kPa (77 mmHg).

11. Your team is treating a patient with acute respiratory distress syndrome (ARDS) associated with pneumonia. He may need ventilation if his condition worsens. His physiology is stable apart from a respiratory rate of 30 per minute. Your boss has asked you to calculate the A–a gradient daily so that his progress can be charted. Yesterday's A–a gradient was 47 kPA. Today he is breathing 60% oxygen and his arterial blood gases show: pH 7·35, $PaCO_2$ 5·6 kPa (43 mmHg), bicarbonate 22.5 mmol/l, BE – 1, PaO_2 10·0 kPa (77 mmHg). What is the A–a gradient today?

Self-assessment – discussion

1. The arterial blood gases show a respiratory acidosis with hypoxaemia. Nine per cent of people with an attack of acute severe asthma have respiratory failure; 1% patients with asthma have a fatal or near fatal attack each year. Previous life-threatening attacks increase the risk of death from asthma. Initial management here is to ensure there is no upper airway obstruction, administer the highest concentration of oxygen possible (15 litres per minute via a reservoir bag mask) and treat her breathing with medication to relieve lower airway obstruction. The initial assessment of breathing should include looking for clinical signs of a pneumothorax, which can occur in asthma. The ICU team should be contacted immediately. A large bore intravenous cannula should be inserted and fluid given quickly (for example, 1–2 litres 0·9% saline stat) because the patient is likely to be dehydrated and needs imminent intubation. We can assume she is drowsy because of hypercapnia and hypoxaemia, but a bedside blood glucose estimation followed by a formal neurological examination should be performed once A, B and C are stable.

2. Patients with severe asthma who have just been intubated require long expiratory times because of severe airway

obstruction. This limits the respiratory rate, otherwise stacking or "gas trapping" occurs. The expiratory time can be lengthened by reducing the respiratory rate or decreasing the inspiratory time (by increasing the inspiratory flow rate) or a combination of the two. Suitable settings would be 6–8 breaths per minute with an inspiratory to expiratory ratio of 1:4 or longer. The ventilator should be set to a pressure limit to prevent barotrauma and with peak airway pressures not exceeding 35–40 cm H_2O. This is slightly complicated by the fact that peak pressures in acute severe asthma do not necessarily reflect alveolar pressures but the pressures needed to overcome bronchial obstruction. An appropriate tidal volume should be < 10 ml kg^{-1}. After excluding pneumothorax and volume depletion in this case, consider stacking as a cause of hypotension. The ventilator should be disconnected and the patient allowed to passively exhale – this can take several seconds and a prolonged wheeze can be heard by placing an ear near the end of the endotracheal tube. If this is the cause, the blood pressure will return to normal within seconds. PEEP is not usually of benefit in acute severe asthma as patients already have significant intrinsic or auto-PEEP.

3. The arterial blood gases show a respiratory acidosis with hypoxaemia. Initial management includes an assessment of his airway, medical treatment of his lower airway obstruction, and any other lung pathology that may have triggered his breathlessness (for example, pneumonia or pneumothorax). His oxygen should be increased using a 35% Venturi mask to get the PaO_2 to around 8·0 kPA (60 mmHg). Intravenous fluid should be started for dehydration. If there is no prompt improvement of his respiratory acidosis with medical therapy, non-invasive ventilation should be started. Oxygen therapy is given through the ventilator mask, titrated to arterial blood gases.

4. This man is at risk of further physiological deterioration. He has hypoxaemic respiratory failure despite a high concentration of oxygen. His respiratory rate is 40 per minute. There is also a metabolic acidosis which could indicate hypoperfusion. In this situation, non-invasive CPAP in a critical care area could be tried. This will improve oxygenation and can reduce the work of breathing. However, intubation is indicated within hours if there is no improvement. Intravenous fluids should be administered to treat hypoperfusion, improve oxygen delivery, and aid the expectoration of secretions.

5. The arterial blood gases show a respiratory acidosis with hypoxaemia. Postoperative chest infections and respiratory failure often involve atelectasis (owing to the effects of supine position, general anaesthesia, and difficulty in taking a deep breath from poor pain relief). Retained secretions may be the result of an inability to cough properly. Therefore, close attention should be paid to improving analgesia to allow deep breaths and proper coughing. The acute pain team can be consulted, who may

suggest epidural analgesia. Physiotherapy also has an important role to play and in some cases acute physiotherapy can significantly improve respiratory function. Humidified oxygen therapy is indicated in this circumstance as this aids the expectoration of secretions. The oxygen concentration should be increased. Antibiotics should be commenced and blood and sputum cultures sent. If these measures do not help, the ICU should be contacted for advice on further respiratory support.

6. There is a respiratory acidosis. This patient needs intubation both to support ventilation and to protect the airway from aspiration because of the profound muscle weakness seen in patients with Guillain–Barré syndrome. Up to 30% patients with this syndrome admitted to hospital require mechanical ventilation. There is evidence of ventilatory failure (high $PaCO_2$ and increased respiratory rate) as a result of increasing respiratory muscle weakness as indicated by the falling FVC. Closer examination may reveal a patient who is using accessory respiratory muscles and has a cough, which is bovine in nature. Neurological examination may reveal poor bulbar function. Monitoring oxygen saturations and arterial blood gases in this condition are of little help when deciding when to institute respiratory support. Arterial blood gases follow the condition rather than precede it. Autonomic neuropathy can accompany Guillain–Barré syndrome, leading to tachycardia and hypotension, which also require close observation, especially during anaesthesia and intubation, which can precipitate an asystolic cardiac arrest from profound vagal stimulation. Plasmapheresis is useful in severe or rapidly progressing cases.

7. The arterial blood gases show a mixed respiratory and metabolic acidosis with a lower than expected PaO_2. After his airway has been assessed and oxygen increased to 15 litres per minute, the breathing and circulation are treated in the following way: preload is reduced by sitting the patient up and giving small doses of intravenous diamorphine. Frusemide is a pulmonary vasodilator as well as a diuretic and has a quick onset of action in acute severe left ventricular failure. Around 1 mg kg^{-1} frusemide is given in the first instance and an intravenous nitrate infusion (a vasodilator) can be commenced, titrated to effect and blood pressure. If the patient does not improve, a further dose of frusemide ($1–2 \text{ mg kg}^{-1}$) is administered. After this, non-invasive CPAP is indicated to improve both left ventricular and respiratory function. This is appropriate in alert patients with a moderate respiratory acidosis. If the patient deteriorates or fails to improve, intubation is indicated.

8. The airway is fine, as the patient is alert and talking. Breathing and circulation are abnormal. She is extremely breathless but the chest x ray film is normal and the chest sounds clear. Is this because of shock alone? Her arterial blood gases show a lower than expected PaO_2 (the A–a gradient is 41·2 assuming an FiO_2

of 0·6) and a metabolic acidosis from hypoperfusion. The diagnosis is massive pulmonary embolism. Treatment is to give a high concentration of oxygen (for example, 15 litres per minute via a reservoir bag mask), fluid challenges, and thrombolysis. Intravenous thrombolysis should be considered in pulmonary embolism causing shock and is as effective as surgical embolectomy. Newer literature suggests thrombolysis is safe and effective in "sub-massive" pulmonary embolism as well.

9. The arterial blood gases show a severe respiratory acidosis with a metabolic acidosis and hypoxaemia. Management is to secure the airway by intubation, administer enough oxygen to get the PaO_2 to around 8·0 kPA (62 mmHg), treat his exacerbation of COPD and any precipitating infection, and give intravenous fluid. Breathless patients who have been unwell for a few days are often dehydrated and general anaesthesia can cause vasodilatation which also leads to hypovolaemia. This patient has a base deficit of − 4 suggesting hypoperfusion. An unresponsive patient is not appropriate for non-invasive ventilation. However, before the patient is intubated, further information should be sought as to the severity of the patient's chronic lung disease. Has a discussion already taken place about intubation and ventilation between the patient and his specialist? Do the next of kin have information about what the patient would want in these circumstances? What was his quality of life beforehand and what is his anticipated quality of life after potential discharge from ICU?

10. A–a gradient in kPA = 20 − (3·5/0·8) − 10 = 5.0. This is above normal for this patient – this could indicate a pulmonary embolism given the history.

11. A–a gradient in kPA = 0·6 × 95 − (5·6/0·8) − 10·0 = 40. His physiology is stable, the $PaCO_2$ is satisfactory and the A–a gradient is improving rather than worsening.

Further reading

Appadu BL, Hanning CD. Respiratory physiology. In: Pinnock C, Lin T, Smith T (eds). *Fundamentals of Anaesthesia*. London: Greenwich Medical Media Ltd, 1999.

Confalonieri M, Potena A, Carbone G, Della Porta R, Tolley E, Meduri GU. Acute respiratory failure in patients with severe community-acquired pneumonia. A prospective randomised evaluation of non-invasive ventilation. *Am J Respir Crit Care Med* 1999;**160**:1585–91.

Doherty MJ, Greenstone MA. Survey of non-invasive ventilation (NIPPV) in patients with acute exacerbations of chronic obstructive pulmonary disease (COPD) in the UK. *Thorax* 1998;**53**:863–6.

Konstantinides S, Geibel A, Heusel G, Heinrich F, Kasper W. Heparin and alteplase compared with heparin alone in patients with submassive pulmonary embolism. *New Engl J Med* 2002;**347**:1143–50.

Nava S, Ambrosino N, Clini E *et al.* Non-invasive mechanical ventilation in the weaning of patients with respiratory failure due to chronic obstructive pulmonary disease. A randomised controlled trial. *Ann Intern Med* 1998;**128**:721–8.

Plant PK, Owen JL, Elliot MW. The YONIV trial. A multicentre randomised controlled trial of the early use of non-invasive ventilation for acute exacerbations of chronic obstructive pulmonary disease on general respiratory wards. *Lancet* 2000;**355**:1931–5.

Symonds AK (ed). *Non invasive respiratory support.* London: Arnold, 2001.

http://www.brit-thoracic.org.uk/pdf/NIV.pdf

5: Fluid balance and volume resuscitation

By the end of this chapter you will be able to:
- calculate a patient's normal fluid requirements
- understand how fluid balance is affected by illness
- understand the concept of the "third space" and capillary leak
- understand the principles of volume resuscitation
- know about the different types of fluid available including blood
- apply this to your clinical practice

The main aim of fluid therapy in critical illness is to restore tissue perfusion and optimise organ function by correcting hypovolaemia.

Normal fluid requirements

Normal people balance their daily intake and output. Adults exchange approximately 5% of their body water each day. Normal maintenance fluid requirements are calculated as follows:

- 4 ml kg^{-1} per hour for the first 10 kg
- 2 ml kg^{-1} per hour for the second 10 kg
- 1 mg kg^{-1} per hour after that.

So a 70 kg man requires 2640 ml per day – which is where the commonly used 3 litres a day comes from (Table 5.1). Maintenance fluid covers insensible losses plus the required intake to maintain normal fluid balance (like replacing urine output). Insensible losses include things like sweating and breathing and are around 1200 ml per day. The maximum concentrating power of the kidney is 1200 mosmol kg^{-1} so a minimum of 500 ml urine is needed to excrete the daily solute load of 600 mosmol. Oliguria is defined as a urine output of

Table 5.1 Maintenance fluid according to weight

Weight (kg)	ml per hour	ml per 24 hours
50	90	2169
60	100	2400
70	110	2640
80	120	2880
90	130	3120
100	140	3360

< 0·5 ml kg^{-1} per hour for two consecutive hours or < 400 ml in 24 hours. The elderly have a reduced ability to concentrate urine because of age-related nephron loss.

Electrolytes are needed as well as water: 50–150 mmol sodium and 20–40 mmol potassium is the average daily requirement. An average water and sodium requirement can be found in 1 litre 0·9% saline and 2 litres 5% dextrose per 24 hours; however, note that this is maintenance fluid in a normal person.

Accurate replacement of fluid depends on understanding the distribution of water, sodium, and colloid in the body (Figure 5.1). Humans are 60% water. Females have less because of more fat (which contains less water). Total body water is up to 80% in neonates falling to 45% in the elderly. Two-thirds of total body water is in cells (ICF) and the remaining one-third is in the extracellular compartment (ECF). Sodium is the major extracellular cation and, with chloride, provides the effective osmolality (or tonicity) of this compartment. Potassium and phosphate are the major intracellular ions (Table 5.2). The ICF and ECF are separated by a semi-permeable membrane, which allows free movement of water. Movement of sodium and glucose results in movement of water between the ICF and ECF.

Serum osmolality is regulated by osmoreceptors in the hypothalamus. Osmolality is a measure of the total number of particles in a given weight of plasma. Any minor increase (> 2%) is sensed by these receptors and this causes the release of antidiuretic hormone (ADH), which acts on receptors in the collecting duct, opening aquaporin channels and causing water reabsorption with the excretion of a concentrated urine. A reduction in serum osmolality normally inhibits the release of ADH leading to more dilute urine. A normal 70 kg man

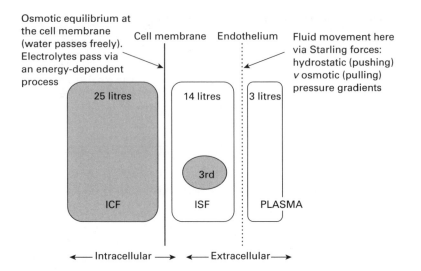

Figure 5.1 Water distribution in the body (of a 70 kg man). Sodium changes in the extracellular compartments cause water shifts to and from cells, contracting or expanding the ICF. The third space is a non-exchangeable compartment in the ISF

Table 5.2 Electrolyte contents of different body compartments (in mmol litre^{-1})

Compartment	Sodium	Potassium	Chloride	Bicarbonate
Plasma	142	4	103	27
Interstitial	144	4	114	30
Intracellular	10	150	0	10

filters 140 litres of water at the glomerulus per day and the majority (70%) is reabsorbed in the proximal convoluted tubule. ADH is controlled to a lesser extent by baroreceptors located in the heart and great vessels. In the presence of volume contraction, ADH is released.

Fluid requirements in illness

Trauma and illness alter the volume and composition of the intracellular and extracellular spaces as well as the kinetics of fluid distribution and excretion. Patients may have increased fluid losses from fever, dehydration, polyuria, bleeding, or breathlessness. An extra 500 ml/day is required for every degree Celsius above 37. Gastrointestinal losses also need to be considered – a patient with diarrhoea or gastric outflow obstruction could be litres behind in terms of fluid balance. Certain patients are at increased risk of pulmonary oedema. Patients with heart failure, renal failure and the elderly are the most common examples. Patients with capillary leak, for example, in severe sepsis, are also at risk of interstitial oedema, yet can require large amounts of intravenous fluid as they are volume depleted. Monitoring and management in these cases is more complex (see Chapter 7).

To preserve plasma volume after trauma, surgery, haemorrhagic shock, or severe sepsis, the kidney reabsorbs filtered water and sodium avidly via ADH. Intravascular volume loss stimulates the renin–angiotensin–aldosterone axis and inhibits natriuretic peptide. This leads to sodium retention (Figure 5.2). Sodium loading occurs with sodium containing crystalloids or colloids. This results in a hyperosmolar state which in turn stimulates further ADH release and fluid retention. This tends to reduce urine output. In addition, high chloride levels from sodium chloride infusions cause renal vasoconstriction and a hyperchloraemic metabolic acidosis. The critically ill have a reduced renal concentrating ability and need to excrete more water to get rid of their solute load. However, these patients often become fluid overloaded and are subsequently fluid restricted, making the problem of sodium retention worse.

To get round these problems of sodium overload in critical illness one should always aim to give specific fluids for specific reasons:

- for electrolyte losses or maintenance – Hartmann's
- for water losses – 5% dextrose or water via nasogastric feeding
- for volume expansion – blood or another appropriate colloid.

Sodium abnormalities in illness

Regulation of salt and water homeostasis is frequently abnormal in hospitalised patients. Hyponatraemia (< 130 mmol litre^{-1}) is the most common electrolyte abnormality

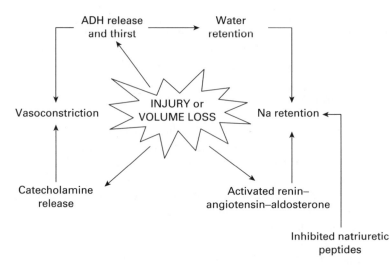

Figure 5.2 Sodium/water retention following surgery or hypovolaemia

with an incidence of 2·5% in the general hospital population. Except in rare circumstances (for example, hyperglycaemia) a reduced serum sodium usually indicates a low serum osmolality and an expanded ICF.

Acute hyponatraemia, defined as a fall in serum Na below 130 mmol litre^{-1} in 48 hours, can result in cerebral oedema. This phenomenon has been described in both adults and children and has been frequently associated with the administration of hypotonic intravenous fluids in the perioperative period. In an adult series of patients having minor surgery, otherwise fit and healthy women were given an average of 8·8 litres in 48 hours – with a net positive balance of 7·5 litres. These patients failed to mount a normal physiological response to expansion of the ECF, which is to produce dilute urine. This is because ADH secretion is increased by a variety of stimuli in hospitalised patients including pain, anxiety, opiate and anaesthetic agents, surgery, and positive pressure ventilation.

The use of hypotonic solutions has been standard in paediatrics for many years and is based on assumptions extrapolated from studies of water requirement and energy expenditure done on normal children almost 50 years ago. The formulae are used for calculating what are commonly referred to as maintenance fluid requirements and this can result in the administration of large amounts of electrolyte-free water (EFW), which then requires the patient to inhibit ADH secretion and produce a dilute urine. Failure to do so would result in a fall in serum sodium with occasionally catastrophic results. The flaw in the application of these formulae is that hospitalised patients do not necessarily follow the rules that govern normal physiology. Different rules apply to sick patients. The assumption should be that when serum sodium is < 140 mmol litre^{-1} in the absence of sodium loss, ADH is acting. These patients, whatever their age, should not be given hypotonic fluids; 4% dextrose/0·18% saline is isotonic before administration but is effectively hypotonic in the patient once the glucose has been metabolised.

A study of over 100 children admitted to hospital with the usual spectrum of medical illnesses showed elevated ADH levels and low serum sodium levels at the time of admission, compared with a cohort of elective surgical admissions who had normal ADH and sodium levels. Other groups particularly at risk for the development of acute hyponatraemia are elderly females treated with thiazide diuretics for hypertension who undergo hip replacement surgery and patients undergoing colonoscopy.

At present the standard of care in many institutions is to use only isotonic fluids during surgery and in the postoperative period. This reduces the risk of a fall in serum sodium. In a study where only Ringer's lactate was used during elective surgery and in the first postoperative day, sodium fell from 140 to 136 mmol litre^{-1}. This was associated with a total intravenous intake of 5 litres and a positive balance of 3 litres. The explanation for this fall despite isotonic fluids was demonstrated when urine sodium was measured. Most of the patients were producing a hypertonic urine (sodium > 150 mmol litre^{-1}). The hypothesis proposed to explain this was that large volumes of fluid were infused during surgery to maintain blood pressure, which falls due to the vasodilatory effect of anaesthetic drugs. When vasomotor tone was restored to normal at the end of surgery, the ECF was overfilled and the kidneys responded by eliminating sodium. In summary, hypotonic fluids may be used when the plasma sodium is > 145 mmol litre^{-1} and there is a need for EFW. Patients with sodium levels < 140 mmol litre^{-1} should receive isotonic fluids.

Capillary leak and the concept of the "third space"

Oedema is excessive fluid accumulation in the interstitial space and can be localised or generalised. Third space losses occur when fluid accumulates in a potential space such as the peritoneum, pleura, or bowel. The concept of the third space was developed to explain the phenomenon that some postoperative patients required more replacement fluid than their measurable losses. Studies showed that the patients' weight did not reduce but that they were intravascularly volume depleted. This was due to movement rather than loss of fluid.

"Capillary leak syndrome" has been defined as a syndrome characterised by a prolonged and severe increase in capillary permeability, the clinical features of which include hypoalbuminaemia, microalbuminuria, severe positive fluid balance, clinical oedema, and decreased oxygen delivery and uptake.

Capillary leak or microvascular failure is part of the inflammatory response to a range of insults (Figure 5.3). Studies have shown rapid and profound transcapillary loss of radiolabelled albumin occurring within 6 hours of surgery and similar changes occur in patients with severe inflammatory conditions (for example, sepsis, trauma, and ischaemia). The kidneys are uniquely placed to mirror changes in capillary permeability because they receive 25% of the cardiac output, which is filtered over a wide surface area. The unique nature of the renal-concentrating mechanism allows low level albumin loss (microalbuminuria) to be used as a sensitive monitor of changes in systemic capillary permeability. In uncomplicated cases capillary permeability returns to normal within 24 hours of major surgery. In extreme cases the result is SIRS – systemic inflammatory response syndrome – an unregulated inflammatory response that results in significant end-organ dysfunction and later multiple organ dysfunction syndrome (MODS) (Figure 5.4).

Haemorrhagic shock

Blood volume is normally 7% body weight (5 litres in a 70 kg man). Acute loss of circulating blood leads to compensatory

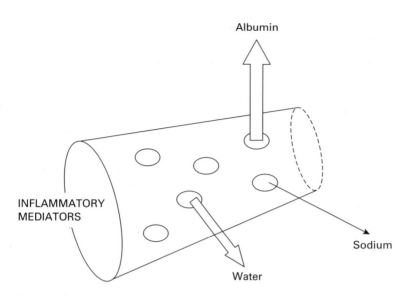

Figure 5.3 Capillary leak after major surgery or in critical illness. Electron microscopy in rats with severe sepsis shows holes that appear in the endothelium

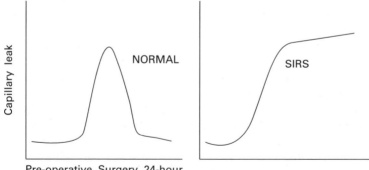

Figure 5.4 Microalbuminuria as a measure of capillary leak during surgery and in systemic inflammatory response syndrome (SIRS)

responses. Tachycardia is the first measurable sign. At the cellular level, inadequately perfused cells compensate initially by anaerobic metabolism producing a lactic acidosis. Mild metabolic acidosis is common following major surgery for this

Table 5.3 Estimated fluid and blood losses based on patient's initial presentation (for a 70 kg man)

Losses	Class 1	Class 2	Class 3	Class 4
Blood loss (ml)	Up to 750	750–1500	1500–2000	Over 2000
Blood loss or tennis score (% blood vol)	Up to 15% loss	15–30% loss	30–40% loss	Over 40% loss
Pulse rate	< 100	> 100	> 120	> 140
Blood pressure	Normal	Normal	Reduced	Reduced
Pulse pressure*	Normal	Reduced	Reduced	Reduced
Respiratory rate	14–20	20–30	30–40	> 35
Urine output (ml h^{-1})	> 30	20–30	5–15	Negligible
CNS	Alert	Mild anxiety	Anxious and confused	Confused and lethargic

*Pulse pressure is the difference between systolic and diastolic blood pressure. (Adapted with permission from the American College of Surgeons: Committee on Trauma. *Advanced Trauma Life Support for Doctors. Student course manual.* 6th edn. Chicago: American College of Surgeons, 1997.)

reason and a persistent metabolic acidosis in some patients may indicate inadequate fluid resuscitation. Eventually cell membrane damage and cell swelling occurs which leads to fluid shifts. The best way to think of haemorrhage is by using tennis scores (Table 5.3).

By the time blood pressure has dropped in a healthy patient because of bleeding, at least 30% of circulating blood volume has been lost. Certain groups do not manifest the usual signs of hypovolaemia: athletes can compensate for blood loss very well, patients on beta blockers or calcium antagonists may not generate a tachycardia, and patients with permanent pacemakers and the elderly also have altered responses. Therefore a 30% loss of blood volume (nearly 2 litres in an average adult) is the smallest amount of blood loss that consistently causes a drop in systolic blood pressure – classical haemorrhagic shock.

Fluid resuscitation

Successful fluid resuscitation is integral to the management of the critically ill patient. However, volume status can sometimes be difficult to assess. This makes it vitally important to have an effective strategy to define both trigger points to institute therapy and endpoints when the goal of therapy has been reached. Trigger points are based on a thorough assessment of the patient including history and examination. History alone can point to likely hypovolaemia, for example bowel obstruction, sepsis, burns, pancreatitis, and trauma. Markers of inadequate circulating volume include:

Skin temperature

Cold extremities can be a sign of poor organ perfusion. A capillary refill time of more than 2 seconds is significant. The central–peripheral temperature gradient has long been used in surgical specialties as an early warning sign for hypovolaemia. When the difference between core (nasopharynx or tympanic) and peripheral (great toe) temperature increases, it is due to vasoconstriction. This can be a sign of hypovolaemia although pain, vasoactive drugs and central hypothermia are confounding variables.

One study looked at whether physical examination alone in combination with biochemical markers could accurately diagnose hypoperfusion: 264 consecutive surgical intensive care patients were divided into two groups – those with cool extremities and those with warm extremities. Vital signs, arterial blood gases and lactate, haemoglobin, and PA catheter data were collected from these patients. There was no difference between the two groups with regard to heart rate, systolic blood pressure, pulmonary arterial occlusion pressure, haemoglobin, PaO_2, or $PaCO_2$. However cardiac output and pH were significantly lower in the cool extremity patients compared with the warm extremity patients. The investigators concluded that combining physical examination with serum bicarbonate and lactate readily identified patients with hypoperfusion.

Respiratory rate

Respiratory rate increases in hypoperfusion as the body tries to compensate by increasing oxygen delivery and increasing the removal of acid waste products. Respiratory rate increases in early haemorrhage and a rate of above 20 breaths per minute is significant.

Metabolic (lactic) acidosis

Of patients requiring ICU admission, 57% present with a metabolic acidosis and, in three-quarters of these, it is due to a raised lactate because of hypoperfusion. A raised lactate is associated with increased mortality. A base deficit of more than -4 mmol litre^{-1} on admission to the ICU is associated with an in-hospital mortality of 57%, which rises to 70% if it is not corrected within 24 hours. The base deficit has been shown to correlate with intravascular fluid requirements in patients with trauma.

Reduced conscious level

Cerebral blood flow is autoregulated between mean blood pressure values of 60–150 mmHg. A reduction in cerebral perfusion pressure leads to drowsiness, confusion, irritability, and finally coma.

Orthostatic blood pressure measurements

Blood pressure can be "normal" in elderly or normally hypertensive patients with hypovolaemia. Whilst supine hypotension implies significant blood volume loss, young people can compensate well and 30% of the elderly have postural hypotension as an incidental finding.

Urine output

When any patient becomes oliguric, perfusion should be assessed. Oliguria can be a sign that the patient is deteriorating.

As vital signs such as blood pressure and pulse can be unhelpful, multiple clinical variables must be assessed in order to gain an overall picture when deciding on volume status. No one variable should be taken in isolation. If there is any uncertainty about volume status, a fluid challenge is the safest way to assess this further. The fluid challenge is a fundamental manoeuvre – the aim is to produce a small but rapid increase in plasma volume and then to assess the response.

The physiological relationship between cardiac filling and cardiac output is described in Starling's curve (see Figure 6.1, p 106). This curve describes the functional consequences of alterations in preload on cardiac output and is the rationale behind improving cardiac output with volume administration. Up to a certain point, volume expansion leads to an increased cardiac output owing to increased end-diastolic ventricular filling. Beyond this, increased end-diastolic volume will lead to a reduced cardiac output. Measurement of cardiac responses in response to a fluid challenge can therefore be used to define optimal filling pressures (Figure 5.5). A suitable fluid challenge is 250 ml colloid over 10 minutes. This may need to be repeated.

Colloids are effective volume expanders for resuscitation, especially in situations where changes in capillary permeability have occurred. Different colloids have different properties. Crystalloids are isotonic and rapidly distribute throughout the extracellular space causing oedema. Crystalloids also have to be given in large volumes to achieve significant volume expansion: 1000 ml of 0·9% sodium chloride would increase the plasma volume by 200 ml and be short-lived.

It is also important to understand that simply speeding up maintenance fluid is not an effective way to treat volume depletion, as shown in Figure 5.6. The increased maintenance fluid could take hours to make a patient euvolaemic. During this time hypoperfusion could cause irreversible renal damage and metabolic acidosis – problems that become more difficult to correct with time.

A fluid challenge should be given through a large bore cannula (14–16G) and wide diameter giving set to give an adequate flow rate (Table 5.4).

A triple lumen central venous catheter has different sized ports – the largest is designed for fluid and the others for measurement and infusions. The relatively small diameter and long length of a central line compared with a 14G cannula makes it less suitable for resuscitation when fluid needs to be given quickly.

Assessment of the fluid challenge can be either pressure-based (for example, blood pressure and CVP) or flow-based (for example, cardiac output measurements). When pressure based, a common approach is to continue giving boluses of fluid until a sustained rise in central venous pressure (CVP) occurs, rather

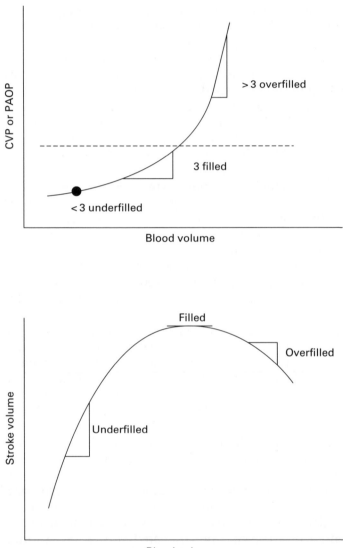

Figure 5.5 The response of CVP/PAOP and stroke volume to small volume fluid challenges. In a hypovolaemic patient, an increase in stroke volume with no significant rise in CVP/PAOP would be expected. In the optimally filled patient, a rise in CVP/PAOP with no significant rise in stroke volume would be expected. CVP, central venous pressure; PAOP, pulmonary artery occlusion pressure

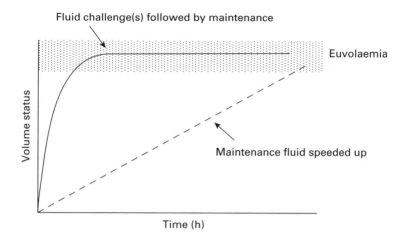

Figure 5.6 The effect of fluid challenge(s) versus maintenance fluids

Table 5.4 Flow rates and diameters of cannulae

Size of cannula	Colour code	Flow rate (ml min⁻¹)
24G	Yellow	18
22G	Blue	36
20G	Pink	61
18G	Green	90
16G	Grey	200
14G	Brown	300

than be limited by a predetermined value. A normal heart rate, blood pressure, and CVP do not exclude volume depletion and a single CVP reading is unreliable in assessing volume status. The "rule of threes" is a more useful tool. If the CVP increases by 3 mmHg and then falls back to the original value after 5 minutes, a further fluid challenge should be administered. If the CVP increases by 3 mmHg and remains elevated, no further fluid is indicated. If the CVP increases by more than 3 mmHg and is above 10 mmHg, the patient could be overfilled. However there is no "normal" CVP and initial measurements greater than 10 mmHg are common and can be due to reasons other than volume status (see Chapter 6).

Some patients continue to show signs of inadequate perfusion (cold extremities, increased respiratory rate, metabolic acidosis, and oliguria) despite an apparently optimal intravascular volume. Early referral to the ICU is required as more advanced monitoring and treatment with vasoactive drugs may be necessary. Pulmonary artery catheters, oesophageal Doppler, and other flow-based monitors permit measurement of cardiac output and other derived measurements, such as systemic vascular resistance, so that predefined oxygen delivery goals may be achieved.

Different types of fluid

Crystalloids

Crystalloids are substances that form a true solution and pass freely through semipermeable membranes. They contain water, dextrose, and electrolytes, and stay in the intravascular compartment for about 45 minutes.

Crystalloids pass easily through capillary and glomerular membranes but, although they do not diffuse through cell membranes, membrane pumps and metabolism soon alter their distribution. Their composition varies depending on the type of solution. Sodium is the particle responsible for plasma volume expansion and this determines the initial distribution of the crystalloid (isotonic solutions will distribute throughout the ECF where sodium is found, but hypotonic solutions, which contain more water, will distribute in cells as well). Dextrose in water is basically free water as it does not contain sodium, and distributes to both the intracellular fluid and extracellular fluid. Dextrose is not an effective plasma expander as inadequate amounts reach the intravascular compartment, and it should never be used in volume resuscitation.

Infusion of 0·9% saline or colloids suspended in 0·9% saline can produce a dose-dependent hyperchloraemic metabolic acidosis. The serum sodium is often normal. Calculation of the anion gap is useful as it is normal in a hyperchloraemic metabolic acidosis but raised in lactic acidosis. The urinary chloride will be high in the former and low in the latter. The clinical significance of saline-induced hyperchloraemic metabolic acidosis is unknown.

Crystalloids are used to restore extracellular electrolyte and volume deficits, are well tolerated, and are usually administered peripherally. Other advantages of crystalloids include low cost, safety, easy storage, and availability. The primary limitation of crystalloids as replacement solutions is the amount of fluid needed to replace plasma volume. It is estimated that 5 litres of crystalloid would replace 1 litre of blood because only one-fourth of the volume reaches the circulation. Using crystalloids as volume expanders has theoretical disadvantages. The subsequent increase in interstitial volume could impair wound healing and gas exchange. The most commonly used crystalloids are:

- sodium chloride 0·9%
- dextrose 5%
- dextrose 4% saline 0·18%
- Hartmann's solution – resembles the extracellular fluid. (Alexis Hartmann was a US paediatrician. Hartmann's solution was used in sick children with a metabolic acidosis because the lactate is metabolised to bicarbonate within a few hours. It is avoided in certain patients: renal failure because of the risk of hyperkalaemia, liver failure because of the risk of lactic acidosis, and diabetes because of lactate metabolism to glucose. The calcium content of Hartmann's means that it may form clots if mixed with stored blood (which contains citrate) in the same intravenous line.)

The electrolyte content of common crystalloids in mmol litre^{-1} (mg dL^{-1}) is shown in Table 5.5.

Colloids

Definition: colloids are substances that do not form true solutions and do not pass through semipermeable membranes. Colloid infusions increase osmotic pressure, draining water out of the interstitial space into the intravascular compartment. They stay in the intravascular compartment for varying lengths of time depending on their molecular weight.

Different colloids have very different properties. The most commonly used colloids are:

Table 5.5 Contents of common crystalloids in mmol litre^{-1} (mg dl^{-1})

Crystalloids	Na$_2^+$	K$^+$	Ca$_2^+$	Cl$^-$	HCO$_3^-$	Osmolality	pH	Other
Plasma	140	4	2·3 (9·2)	100	26	285–295	7·0	
Sodium chloride 0·9%	154	0	0	154	0	308	5·0	
Sodium chloride 0·45%	77	0	0	77	0	154	5·0	
Sodium chloride 3%	513	0	0	513	0	1026	5·0	
Dextrose 5%	0	0	0	0	0	252	4·0	Dextrose 50 g l^{-1}
Dextrose 4% saline 0·18%	30	0	0	0	0	255	4·0	Dextrose 40 g l^{-1}
Hartmann's	131	5	2 (8)	111	29	278	6·5	29 lactate
Ringer's lactate	147	4	2·2 (8·8)	156	0	302		28 lactate
Sodium bicarbonate 1·26%	150	0	0	0	150	300	8	
Sodium bicarbonate 8·4%	1000	0	0	0	1000	2000	8	

- Gelatines (for example, Gelofusine and Haemaccel) – gelatine is a degradation product of animal collagen and is inexpensive and readily available. Different brands vary in electrolyte content. The calcium content of Haemaccel means that it may form clots if mixed with stored blood (which contains citrate) in the same intravenous line.
- Dextrans – these are glucose polymers available in different molecular weights (for example, Dextran 70 = 70 000 Daltons). These are rarely used because of side effects.
- Hydroxyethyl starch (HES) – this is derived from amylopectin, a plant polymer and contains no electrolytes. Unmodified starch is unsuitable as a plasma substitute since it is broken down rapidly by amylase. The hydroxyethylation of starch protects the polymer against breakdown. Different products with different mean molecular weights exist. Larger particles have a higher degree of protection from metabolism and give a more prolonged effect (days). HES is therefore useful in patients with capillary leak. Some research suggests that HES reduces capillary leak by an unknown mechanism. It cannot be used alone if greater than 30% plasma volume replacement is needed – water should be given as well, otherwise an osmotic nephrosis and acute renal failure can occur.
- Human albumin solution (HAS) – albumin is the fraction of plasma that provides the main part of the circulation's osmotic pressure and has therefore been used as a plasma substitute. It is derived from human plasma and is heat sterilised so it is virtually disease-free; 4.5% HAS reflects normal plasma; 20% HAS has water and salt removed – hence it is sometimes called "salt-poor albumin". HAS was mainly used to replace fluid losses in burns where high albumin loss is also a problem. The major limitations to the use of HAS are high production costs and limited supplies. Albumin has a number of other functions which include:

  - transport of molecules
  - free radical scavenging
  - binding of toxins
  - inhibition of platelet aggregation.

Colloids are either monodispersed like albumin if the molecular size and weight are uniform throughout the product, or polydispersed if there are a variety of different molecular sizes and shapes like starches. The molecular weight determines the retention time and duration of colloidal effect in the circulation. Lower molecular weight particles have a higher osmotic effect but are rapidly excreted by the kidneys in contrast to larger particles.

Most colloid solutions are subject to maximum limits suggested by the manufacturers on the basis of available research data. Most UK colloids are suspended in sodium chloride but colloids in 5% dextrose are available in the USA.

The retention of both crystalloids and colloids in the circulation is variable. In dehydration, retention time may be increased but, in critical illness with its associated capillary leak, retention times are shorter. Generally, crystalloids stay in the circulation for less than an hour. Gelatines stay in the circulation for a few hours. Albumin has two half lives, the first being only 4 hours. Starch solutions have a half life of several days.

Allergic phenomena and coagulation abnormalities with colloids

Allergic reactions range from urticaria, the most common effect of gelatines, to severe anaphylaxis with cardiovascular collapse, more commonly seen with dextrans. The incidence of allergic reactions is low with any of the colloids (0·01%–0·05%).

Colloids affect coagulation through various mechanisms but these effects are rarely associated with clinical bleeding:

- A dilution coagulopathy is associated with any plasma substitute.
- Dextrans reduce the activities of factor V and VIII. These effects are more severe with higher molecular weights.
- Gelatines interfere with fibrin polymerisation and inhibit platelet aggregation.
- HES solutions interfere with Von Willebrand and factor VIII release and accelerates the conversion of fibrinogen to fibrin, which results in weaker clot formation.

Table 5.6 Contents and anaphylaxis rate of common colloids in mmol litre^{-1} (mg dl^{-1})

Colloids	Na$_2^+$	K$^+$	Ca$_2^+$	Cl$^-$	Osmolality	pH	Duration of volume effect*	Anaphylaxis (%)
Plasma	140	4	2·3 (9·2)	100	285–295	7·0		
Gelofusine	154	0·4	0·4 (1·6)	125	279	7·4	1–2 hours	0·345
Haemaccel	145	5·1	6·25 (25)	145	301	7·3	1–2 hours	0·345
Dextran 70	0	0	0	0	287	5·0	1–2 hours	0·273
Albumin 4·5%	145	<2	0	145	290	7·4	2–4 hours	0·099
Albumin 20%	145	<2	0	145	290	7·4	2–4 hours	0·099
HES 6%	0	0	0	0	300	5·5	6–18 hours	0·058
Stored red cells							Several days	

*Varies depending on the volume status of the patient and the presence of capillary leak.

Blood

Giving blood carries a small risk and uses a valuable resource. The trend is more towards giving blood only when absolutely necessary. The following are indications for blood transfusion:

- to expand intravascular volume in serious haemorrhage
- to restore oxygen carrying capacity.

The decision to transfuse blood for anaemia depends very much on volume status, ongoing blood loss, and any pre-existing myocardial or cerebrovascular ischaemia rather than on an absolute haemoglobin. Blood may be required in life-threatening haemorrhage even if the haemoglobin is normal. On the other hand, stable patients can tolerate anaemia well via compensatory mechanisms and consideration of blood transfusion in these patients is usually only appropriate when the Hb falls below 8 g dl^{-1}.

Stored whole blood has a haematocrit of 40% but plasma, platelets, and other components are removed, leaving concentrated red cells with a haematocrit of 60%. It can be stored at 1–6°C for 28 days. Acid citrate dextrose is one of the most common additives to prevent clotting. The acid acts as a buffer, the citrate binds calcium, which inhibits clotting, and the dextrose acts as a substrate for red cells. Platelets reduce to virtually zero after 24 hours of storage and clotting factors V and Vlll are reduced to 50% after 21 days.

- O negative blood is immediately available.
- Type-specific blood (group and rhesus state only) is ready in 5 minutes.
- Fully cross-matched blood is ready in 20 minutes.

The risks of transfusion decrease with more specific matching. Transfusion reactions are rare but can occur with only small amounts of blood. Death occurs in 1 in 100 000 transfusions. Reactions range from fever to haemolytic syndromes, acute renal failure, and anaphylaxis.

Complications of blood transfusion are immunological, infective, metabolic, or general (for example, hypothermia and fluid overload) and there are further complications with large blood transfusions (Box 5.1).

Box 5.1 Complications of blood transfusion.

Immunological
- Haemolysis, immediate or delayed
- Anaphylaxis
- Increased risk of infection and recurrence or cancer postoperatively

Infective
- Rarely, red cells may become contaminated with bacteria during storage. There is rapid development of sepsis and cardiovascular collapse.
- UK blood is screened for hepatitis B and C, HIV-2 and syphilis. Donors undergo rigorous health screening with several exclusion criteria. Since 1998, 95% of white cells are removed because of a theoretical risk of nvCJD transmission.

Metabolic
- Potassium, calcium and acid-base balance may be affected.

Massive blood transfusion (for example, 10 units within 6 hours) has particular problems in addition to those of transfusion generally:

- Coagulopathy
- Hypothermia
- Hypocalcaemia
- Hyperkalaemia
- Metabolic acidosis followed by metabolic alkalosis from citrate
- ARDS (acute respiratory distress syndrome)

Many blood transfusions are given to treat a haemoglobin level rather than the patient. One randomised Canadian study (TRICC) looked at two groups of stable patients in ICU. In the first group, blood transfusion was triggered at a haemoglobin of 7 g dl^{-1} and maintained at 7–9. The second group was transfused if the haemoglobin fell below 10 g dl^{-1} and was maintained at 10–12. There was no advantage for the patients with higher haemoglobins and blood transfusions were reduced by 54% overall. At the time of writing one unit of blood costs £72 in the UK. The TRICC study found a survival advantage in the lower haemoglobin group among certain subgroups of patients. A lower haemoglobin conferred an advantage if the APACHE II score was < 20 and the age was < 55.

A recent study published in the journal *JAMA* looked at blood transfusions in ICUs across Europe. Transfused patients had a significantly higher mortality despite similar disease severity scores. The authors suggested that red cell transfusions may contribute to immunosuppression.

Studies have shown that perioperative blood transfusion increases the risk of infectious complications after major surgery and of cancer recurrence after curative surgery. This is thought to be related to the immunosuppressant effects of allogeneic blood transfusion and the fact that stored blood contains angiogenic factors.

Mini-tutorial: the crystalloid versus colloid debate

Despite much debate concerning the choice of fluid in volume resuscitation, the crystalloid versus colloid debate has largely reached a stalemate. During the World War II, surgeons realised that salt and water are retained after surgery and it became common practice to restrict them. There were subsequent problems with volume depletion because third space losses were not appreciated. In the 1960s studies showed that patients who received crystalloid and blood did better than patients who only received blood. Shire showed in animal experiments, using radioactive tracers, that the interstitial compartment contracts during trauma and major surgery. Crystalloids not only resuscitate the intravascular compartment, they resuscitate this compartment as well, but large volumes of crystalloid are needed to resuscitate the intravascular compartment because they are quickly distributed throughout the ECF – this can lead to problems with interstitial oedema when large amounts of crystalloid are given. With the advent of synthetic colloids, many people believed these were better, because they were more effective at expanding the intravascular compartment. They are faster to give, with less sodium load and risk of hypothermia, and a more rapid expansion in plasma volume restores tissue perfusion quickly, which can prevent tissue damage and the subsequent release of inflammatory mediators. However, allergic reactions can occur and colloids are more expensive. Studies have shown no difference in mortality but the cost per life saved using colloids is much more.

All the studies that have been done comparing crystalloids and colloids have yielded conflicting results. Extensive research has failed to show the superiority of colloids or crystalloids. Most colloid advocates do not recommend colloids as the only fluid to be used in resuscitation. It may be that certain subgroups of patients benefit from one type of fluid over another – but there is no definitive answer and the debate goes on.

Mini-tutorial: controversies over albumin

A recent Cochrane review looked at human albumin administration in the critically ill and its effects on mortality. The results were widely publicised; 30 trials met the inclusion criteria (1419 patients). The investigators found that the risk of death for patients receiving albumin was 14% compared with 8% in controls – or that for every 17 critically ill patients treated with albumin there was one additional death. The validity of the studies included in the systematic review was extensively debated. A later publication pointed out that more than half the trials included were pre-1990 and did not reflect current practice. The trials also included a mixture of patients with different characteristics and many were not blinded. Nevertheless, the debate did spark a controversy and probably contributed to a reduction in albumin use.

Albumin is sometimes given to treat hypoalbuminaemia, which occurs in critical illness. This has not been shown to improve outcome when compared with that for synthetic colloids. Albumin leaks from the circulation in critical illness, but serum albumin levels do not correlate with the osmotic pressure of the intravascular compartment. Studies have shown similar osmotic pressures in critically ill patients with low versus normal albumins. However, albumin administration reduces mortality when given in spontaneous bacterial peritonitis and is also used in the hepatorenal syndrome. None of the controversy around albumin applies to its evidence-based use in liver disease.

Self-assessment – case histories

1. A 60-year-old man returns to the ward, having had a laparotomy for bowel obstruction which lasted 2 hours. You are informed that his urine output for the last 2 hours has been < 30 ml h^{-1}. In theatre he received 1 litre of Hartmann's and 1 litre of Gelofusine. His vital signs are: pulse 80 per minute, blood pressure 140/70 mmHg, respiratory rate 20 per minute, and core temperature 37·5°C. The nurse is concerned about his urine output. How do you assess his volume status?

2. A 55-year-old man is on the coronary care unit when he develops a low urine output (< 0·5 mg kg^{-1} per hour for the last 2 hours). His vital signs are: pulse 90 per minute, blood pressure 110/50 mmHg, respiratory rate 22 per minute, and core temperature 37°C. He has cool hands and feet. He had an inferolateral myocardial infarction 24 hours ago. The nurse is concerned about his urine output. How do you assess his volume status?

3. A young woman arrives in the medical admissions unit with diarrhoea, which she has had for several days. She also has a macular rash and a high fever. She has a systolic blood pressure of 70 mmHg and a pulse of 130 per minute. Her blood tests show an elevated urea and creatinine with low platelets. What is your immediate management?

4. A middle-aged man comes to the Emergency Department having fallen on the path and hurt his left lower ribs. His observations are: pulse 110 per minute and blood pressure 140/90 mmHg. You notice how clammy he feels to touch. Could this man have a life-threatening haemorrhage?

5. An 80-year-old lady is admitted with abdominal pain and malaena. She has a permanent pacemaker and is treated for congestive cardiac failure, which is under control. Her pulse and blood pressure are normal. How can you assess her volume status?

6. A 50-year-old man weighing 70 kg with no past medical history is admitted with gastric outflow obstruction and is scheduled for surgery later in the week. His fluid balance chart for the last 24 hours is as follows. Input: nil orally, 3 litres intravenous 0·9% sodium chloride. Output: urine 500 ml total, bowels nil, nasogastric tube 4000 ml total. There are no intravenous antibiotics or other drugs, and no fever is recorded. This morning's blood results show: Na 150 mmol litre^{-1}, K 3·0 µmol litre^{-1}, urea 12 mmol litre^{-1} (33·3 mg dl^{-1}), creatinine 140 µmol litre^{-1} (1·68 mg dl^{-1}). What fluids should you prescribe for the next 24 hours?

7. A patient comes back from theatre to your high dependency area. His vital signs are: pulse 80 per minute, blood pressure 150/80 mmHg, respiratory rate 25 per minute, and core temperature 36°C. His arterial blood gases show: pH 7·3, PaO_2 15·0 kPa (115 mmHg), $PaCO_2$ 4·0 (29 mmHg) and bicarbonate 14·5 mmol/l, BE – 6. His CVP reading is 12 mmHg. He received Hartmann's and blood in theatre. How do you manage his acidosis?

8. A patient on ICU with a tracheostomy has been on maintenance crystalloid (0·9% saline) for several days and this morning's blood results show: Na 145 mmol litre^{-1}, K 4·0 mmol litre^{-1}, urea 4·5 mmol litre^{-1} (12·5 mg dl^{-1}), creatinine 80 µmol l^{-1} (0·96 mg dl^{-1}). The patient is stable and the vital signs are: pulse 60 per minute, blood pressure 130/65 mmHg, respiratory rate 12 per minute and core temperature 36·5°C. The arterial blood gases show: pH 7·3, PaO_2 13·0 (100 mmHg), $PaCO_2$ 4·5 (34·6 mmHg) and bicarbonate 16·3 mmol/l, BE – 5. The patient is doing well in every way and is expected to leave ICU in the next 24 hours. The examination is normal. Can you explain the arterial blood gas results?

9. You have just put a CVP line into a patient who is unwell with a severe biliary infection. The CVP measures 15 mmHg. What is your next course of action?

10. A postoperative patient's blood results are as follows: Na 120 mmol litre^{-1}, K 4·0 mmol litre^{-1}, urea 6·0 mmol litre^{-1} (16·6 mg dl^{-1}), creatinine 95 µmol l^{-1} (1·14 mg dl^{-1}). How do you assess the low sodium in order to treat it correctly?

Self-assessment – discussion

1. The history alone in this case tells you that the patient is likely to be hypovolaemic – he has a history of bowel obstruction and has just had a laparotomy, so is likely to have a combination of hypovolaemia with capillary leak and interstitial oedema. Check skin temperature and capillary refill at the peripheries as it may be reduced if there is hypovolaemia. His respiratory rate is raised. Arterial blood gases may reveal a base deficit suggesting tissue hypoperfusion. A fluid challenge should be given if there are signs of hypovolaemia or if there is any uncertainty about his volume status. This kind of patient should never be given a diuretic as first-line treatment for a poor urine output. It would be appropriate to give 250 ml colloid over 10 minutes and assess the response.

2. Patients admitted to hospital following a myocardial infarction can be dehydrated due to vomiting, sweating, and reduced oral intake. His respiratory rate is raised and his peripheral skin temperature may be reduced. In this case, you would want to know if there are any crackles audible in the lungs. Arterial blood gases may reveal a base deficit. A fluid challenge can be given safely if there are signs of hypovolaemia or if there is any uncertainty about this patient's volume status. The definition of cardiogenic shock includes a low cardiac output state, which is unresponsive to fluid (see Chapter 6) and this implies that fluid is used in the assessment of this condition.

3. The picture is of a young person with severe sepsis. A search for the focus of infection should take place but this should not take priority over A, B, C, and "blind" antibiotic therapy. After you have initiated high concentration oxygen therapy, two large bore cannulae should be inserted and fluid challenges given. There is a history of diarrhoea for several days, which implies severe volume depletion – but in the context of severe sepsis, an abnormally low systemic vascular resistance means that the hypotension may not respond to fluid alone, and invasive monitoring and vasopressors may be required.

4. Yes. It is highly possible that this man has ruptured his spleen. Airway is okay. Check breathing (for pneumothorax) and insert two large bore cannulae for fluid. Assess capillary refill. He could have lost 20–30% of his circulating blood volume already and needs urgent imaging and surgery.

5. This is exactly the type of patient in whom volume status can be incredibly difficult to assess. The elderly do not respond physiologically to bleeding in the same way as younger patients. The history of a gastrointestinal bleed points to volume depletion, as does chronic diuretic use. Although she has a "normal" blood pressure – is it *her* normal? Special attention must be paid to other markers of hypoperfusion in this lady, as

pulse and blood pressure (including orthostatic measurements) will be of little value. Look at peripheral skin temperature and respiratory rate, and perform an arterial blood gas analysis. A urinary catheter should be inserted to monitor hourly urine output.

6. The blood tests and the fluid balance chart suggest volume depletion. Large nasogastric losses have resulted in hypokalaemia. In a dehydrated patient with hypernatraemia, total body water deficit may be calculated as follows:

$$\text{Volume in litres needed} = 0.5 \times \frac{[Na_2^+] - 140}{140}$$

0·5 is the approximate total body water (TBW). In this patient the TBW deficit is 3·57 litres (Table 5.7). This is required over the next 24 hours in addition to his maintenance requirements and anticipated ongoing nasogastric losses. Hartmann's at 110 ml h^{-1} is appropriate as maintenance fluid; 5% dextrose with additional potassium can replace water losses – 4 litres can be given in addition to the Hartmann's over the next 24 hours.

Table 5.7 Daily volumes and electrolyte contents (mmol litre^{-1}) of body secretions

Body secretions	ml 24 h^{-1}	Na$_2^+$	K$^+$	Cl$^-$	HCO$_3^-$
Saliva	+ 1500	10	25	10	30
Stomach	+ 1500	50	10	130	0
Duodenum	+ 1000	140	5	80	0
Ileum	+ 3000	140	5	104	30
Colon	− 6000	60	30	40	0
Pancreas	+ 500	140	5	75	100
Biliary	+ 500	140	5	100	30
Sweat	+ 1000	50	0	0	0

7. The history tells you that the metabolic acidosis is most likely due to lactate because of hypoperfusion. Other markers of hypoperfusion should be checked – peripheral skin temperature, respiratory rate, and urine output. "Normal" blood pressure, pulse, and CVP readings do not exclude hypovolaemia. Fluid challenges should be given and the response assessed. Patients returning from theatre often have a reduced core temperature and as they rewarm, vasodilatation causes relative hypovolaemia, which requires fluid. A metabolic acidosis that worsens rather than improves with fluid therapy and rewarming suggests a problem in the abdomen (bleeding or ischaemia) which needs urgent investigation.

8. Prolonged infusions of 0·9% sodium chloride can lead to a hyperchloraemic metabolic acidosis. Controversy has surrounded the aetiology and clinical relevance of the acidifying potential of

large volumes of sodium chloride solutions. The term "dilutional acidosis" implies that plasma expansion and a consecutive dilutional reduction of plasma bicarbonate are the underlying mechanisms. In contrast others have suggested the importance of hyperchloraemia resulting in a reduction of the strong ion difference (SID), calculated as [Na] + [K] – [chloride] – [lactate].

9. The next course of action is to treat the patient on the basis of your assessment of volume status, not a single CVP reading. A fluid challenge should be given and the response of the CVP to this assessed. The "rule of threes" can be used.

10. Hyponatraemia results from salt losses alone or salt and water loss with water replacement. There are several causes of hyponatraemia and one should aim to treat the cause rather than simply fluid restricting the patient (Figure 5.7):

After clinical examination, plasma and urine osmolality and sodium levels should be measured.

- Serum osmolality high (> 295 mosm kg^{-1}) – "hypertonic hyponatraemia from hypoglycaemia, mannitol, or glycine irrigation;

- Serum osmolality normal – pseudohyponatraemia;

- Serum osmolality low (<280 mosm kg^{-1}) – "hypotonic hyponatraemia"

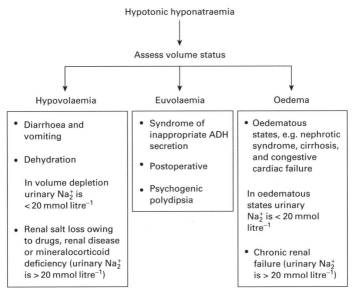

Figure 5.7 Assessment of hyponatraemia

Further reading

Allison KP, Gosling P, Jones S, Pallister I, Porter KM. Randomised trial of hydroxyethyl starch versus gelatine for trauma resuscitation. *J Trauma Injury Infect Crit Care* 1999;**47**:1114–21.

Choi PT, Yip G, Quinonez LG, Cook DG. Crystalloids vs colloids in fluid resuscitation. A systematic review. *Crit Care Med* 1999;**27**:200–10.

Hasibeder WR. Fluid resuscitation during capillary leak. Does the type of fluid make a difference. *Intens Care Med* 2002;**28**:532–4.

Kaplan LJ, McPartland K, Santora TA, Trooskin SZ. Start with a subjective assessment of skin temperature to identify hypoperfusion in ICU patients. *J Trauma Injury Infect Crit Care* 2001;**50**:620–7.

Park GR, Roe PG. *Fluid balance and volume resuscitation for beginners*. London: Medical Media Ltd, 2000.

6: Circulatory failure and the use of inotropes

> **By the end of this chapter you will be able to:**
> - understand what happens in shock
> - understand the basic physiology of the circulation
> - know that pressure is not the same as flow
> - use inotropes logically
> - understand how to use and interpret central venous pressure measurements
> - understand the principles and controversies surrounding the PA catheter
> - be aware of other ways of measuring cardiac output
> - understand the principles of the medical treatment of cardiogenic shock
> - apply this to your clinical practice

Shock

Shock is when the circulation is unable to perfuse and oxygenate the tissues adequately. Hypoperfusion can occur at "normal" blood pressures especially in patients who are usually hypertensive. The markers of inadequate perfusion are discussed in Chapter 5. Traditionally, shock is divided into five types:

- haemorrhagic (see Chapter 5)
- cardiogenic
- septic (see Chapter 7)
- anaphylactic
- neurogenic (after high spinal cord injury due to loss of sympathetic tone).

The characteristic haemodynamic variables in the different types of shock are shown in Table 6.1.

Compensatory mechanisms in shock first aim to restore blood pressure and then intravascular volume. Falling blood

Table 6.1 Characteristic haemodynamic variables in different types of shock

Shock type	CO	SVR	PAOP/CVP
Cardiogenic	▼ ▼	▲	Any
Hypovolaemic	▼	▲ ▲	▼ ▼
Septic	▲ ▲	▼ ▼ ▼	▼ ▼
Anaphylactic	▼	▼ ▼	▼ ▼
Neurogenic	▼	▼ ▼ ▼	▼ ▼

CO, cardiac output; CVP, central venous pressure; PAOP, pulmonary artery occlusion pressure; SVR, systemic vascular resistance

pressure reduces the activity of pressure receptors in the arterial system, which leads to stimulation of the sympathetic nervous system, both centrally and via the adrenal glands. In cardiogenic or hypovolaemic shock, arterial vasoconstriction occurs and blood is diverted to vital organs (for example, the coronary arteries and brain). Tachycardia and vasoconstriction raise the cardiac output. Slower mechanisms aim to restore volume – the lower filtration pressure in the glomerulus activates the renin–angiotensin–aldosterone axis, thirst results, ADH is released because of reduced atrial pressure, and erythropoietin is manufactured.

Physiology of circulation

Blood pressure

Blood pressure does not only depend on intravascular volume. Ohm's law (voltage = current × resistance) has been adapted to demonstrate that blood pressure is the product of cardiac output (CO) and systemic vascular resistance (SVR):

$$BP = CO \times SVR$$

Blood pressure and flow are not the same thing. A low blood pressure does not necessarily mean a low cardiac output – it could be due to a low systemic vascular resistance, or both.

SVR may be thought of as the resistance against which the heart pumps. Vasoconstriction increases SVR whereas vasodilatation reduces it.

Mean arterial pressure (MAP) is the average arterial blood pressure throughout the cardiac cycle. This is produced by integrating a pressure signal for the duration of one cycle. A rough calculation is:

$$\frac{(2 \times \text{diastolic}) + \text{systolic pressure}}{3}$$

Many critical care clinicians prefer using MAP because it is less liable to error owing to measuring techniques; it represents the mean pressure available for perfusing vital organs and is often used in studies.

Cardiac output

Cardiac output depends on the interrelated factors of heart rate (HR) and stroke volume (SV):

$$\text{Cardiac output} = \text{HR} \times \text{SV}$$

Stroke volume is the volume of blood ejected by the ventricle with a single contraction. It can be defined as the difference between end-diastolic and end-systolic volume. SV expressed as a percentage is the ejection fraction. Stroke volume has three major determinants:

- contractility
- preload
- afterload

This basic physiology is clinically important because, in low cardiac output states leading to hypoperfusion, the heart rate, preload, afterload, and then contractility should be addressed – in that order. There is little point in trying to pharmacologically improve the contractility of a heart when it is either too empty or too distended to eject.

Contractility

Contractility is the amount of mechanical work that is done for a given preload and afterload. Factors affecting contractility include are given in Box 6.1.

Box 6.1 Factors affecting contractility

Increased contractility

- Sympathetic stimulation
- Positive inotropic drugs, for example, dobutamine, adrenaline

Reduced contractility

- Parasympathetic stimulation
- Negatively inotropic drugs, for example, β-blockers
- Ischaemia/infarction
- Hypoxaemia
- Acidosis
- Low serum calcium

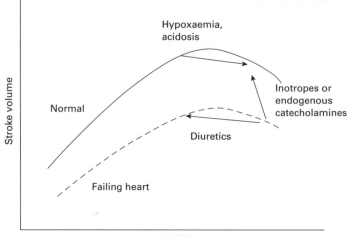

Figure 6.1 The Frank–Starling curve. In isolated myocytes, the tension developed during contraction is dependent on the initial length of the muscle fibre. Laplace's law relates wall tension (T) to internal pressure (P) in an elastic sphere where R is the radius: $P = 2T/R$. Thus, the Frank–Starling relationship for an isolated muscle fibre translates into a relationship between stroke volume and left ventricular end-diastolic pressure (LVEDP)

Preload and afterload

Preload can be defined as the initial length of the muscle fibre before contraction (described by the Frank–Starling curve in Figure 6.1). In a normal heart, we take this to be equivalent

Table 6.2 Receptors in the circulation

Receptor	Action	Where
α receptors	Vasoconstrict	Peripheral, renal, coronary circulation
β1 receptors	Increase contractility, HR, and CO	Heart
β2 receptors	Vasodilate	Peripheral and renal circulation
Dopamine (DA) receptors	Range of actions (see later)	Renal, mesenteric, coronary circulation

CO, cardiac output; HR, heart rate.

to the end-diastolic volume. This is not easily measured. It may be thought of as the filling pressure of the ventricles. In clinical practice the central venous pressure (right ventricle) and pulmonary arterial occlusion pressure (left ventricle) are used to estimate filling pressures – but these have several limitations.

Afterload is defined as the tension developed in the ventricular wall during systole. It is affected by preload, systemic vascular resistance, and external pressure on the ventricles (for example, from positive pressure ventilation). It may be thought of as a measure of how forcefully the ventricles have to contract to eject blood.

Receptors in the circulation

Receptors are important to know about in order to understand how inotropes work. There are four main types of receptor in the circulation (Table 6.2).

All adrenoreceptors act via G proteins and cyclic AMP at the cellular level. Down-regulation of coronary β1 adrenoreceptors occurs in patients who are on long-term β blockers or who have chronic cardiac failure because of prolonged excess endogenous catecholamine release. Down-regulation also occurs with prolonged exogenous catecholamine administration.

Common inotropes

The ideal inotrope would be an agent that increases myocardial contractility in a predictable and easily titratable way without side effects. None exists. Strictly speaking, an inotrope is an agent that increases myocardial contractility whereas a vasopressor is an agent that causes vasoconstriction. A vasoactive drug means either an inotrope or a vasopressor. All should be administered via a central vein.

Dobutamine

Dose range is 1–25 micrograms kg^{-1} per minute. Dobutamine was the first designer inotrope. It has predominant β1 effects, which increase heart rate and contractility and hence cardiac output. It has mild β2 effects, which reduce systemic and pulmonary vascular resistance. Mild α effects may be unmasked in a patient on β blockers. The increase in cardiac work from administration of dobutamine can induce ischaemia in patients with cardiac disease – this is the basis of the dobutamine stress test. However, because of its vasodilatory properties, myocardial oxygen consumption is less than expected because of the reduction in afterload that occurs. These properties make dobutamine a logical first choice inotrope in ischaemic cardiac failure. Dobutamine has no effect on visceral vascular beds; the increased renal and splanchnic flow occur as a resultof increased cardiac output. The increase in cardiac output may increase blood pressure but, since systemic vascular resistance may be reduced or remain unchanged, the effect of dobutamine on systemic blood pressure is variable and depends to some extent on circulatory volume. The indications for and disadvantages of dobutamine are given in Box 6.2.

Box 6.2 Dobutamine indications and disadvantages

Indications

- Low cardiac output states especially if due to ischaemic heart disease

Disadvantages

- May not increase blood pressure
- Tachycardia and arrythmias
- Myocardial ischaemia

Epinephrine (adrenaline)

Dose range is $0.01–0.3$ micrograms kg^{-1} per minute. Epinephrine is a potent β1, β2 and α agonist. The cardiovascular effects of epinephrine depend on dose. At lower doses ($0.005–0.02$ micrograms kg^{-1} per minute which is the equivalent of 1 ml h^{-1} of 5mg epinephrine in 50 ml saline), β1 stimulation predominates, that is, increased contractility, heart rate, and hence cardiac output. There is some stimulation of β2 receptors causing bronchodilation and vasodilatation in certain vascular beds (skeletal muscle). Systemic vascular resistance may fall, which explains the reduction in diastolic blood pressure that is sometimes seen. However, blood pressure tends to rise because β1 effects predominate. Epinephrine also enhances the rate of myocardial relaxation, to allow increased diastolic filling time.

Alpha stimulation becomes more predominant with increasing doses leading to vasoconstriction, which increases systolic blood pressure. There is also visceral bed vasoconstriction at these higher doses. There is a more marked increase in myocardial oxygen consumption than is seen with dobutamine. Other effects include a fall in plasma potassium and a rise in serum glucose. Although its vasoconstrictor effects tend to limit its use, epinephrine is useful in low cardiac output failure unresponsive to dobutamine. This is because increasing cardiac output, but not blood pressure, in severe hypotension may not succeed in improving flow to vital organs that depend on a critical perfusion pressure (the kidneys, coronary arteries, and brain). The indications for and disadvantages of epinephrine are given in Box 6.3.

Box 6.3 Epinephrine (adrenaline) indications and disadvantages

Indications

- Low cardiac output states especially if severe hypotension

Disadvantages

- Tachycardia and arrythmias
- Myocardial ischaemia
- Splanchnic vasoconstriction
- Hypokalaemia and hyperglycaemia

Dopamine

Dose range is 0·5–25 micrograms kg^{-1} per minute. Dopamine stimulates adrenoreceptors and dopaminergic receptors. The effects of dopamine change with increasing dose.

At low doses (up to 3 micrograms kg^{-1} per minute) the predominant effects are those of dopaminergic stimulation causing an increase in renal and mesenteric blood flow. Between doses of 2·5 and 10 micrograms kg^{-1} per minute, β1 receptor effects predominate causing increased myocardial contractility, heart rate, and cardiac output. At doses >10 micrograms kg^{-1} per minute, α stimulation predominates, causing a rise in systemic vascular resistance and reduction in renal blood flow. High doses of dopamine are associated with arrhythmias and increased myocardial oxygen demand.

It has been shown that there is marked individual variation in plasma level compared with dose in the critically ill, making it difficult to know which effects are predominating. Dopamine may accumulate in patients with hepatic dysfunction. There is no evidence to justify using low dose dopamine in acute renal failure either as prevention or treatment (see Chapter 8). The indications for and disadvantages of dopamine are given in Box 6.4.

Box 6.4 Dopamine indications and disadvantages

Indications

- NB No indications for low dose dopamine
- Low cardiac output states

Disadvantages
- Excessive peripheral vasoconstriction
- Tachycardia and arrythmias
- Myocardial ischaemia
- Nausea and vomiting
- Dose does not correspond with blood levels

Dopexamine

Dose range is 0·25–6 micrograms kg^{-1} per minute. Dopexamine is a synthetic analogue of dopamine without α effects. It is a β2 agonist with one-third of the potency of dopamine on DA1 receptors. Dopexamine causes an increase in heart rate and cardiac output as well as causing peripheral vasodilatation and an increase in renal and splanchnic blood flow. Cardiac output is increased as a result of afterload reduction and mild inotropy. In comparison to other inotropes, dopexamine causes less increase in myocardial oxygen consumption. Dopexamine may have some anti-inflammatory activity, but its main focus of interest has been on its ability, at doses of 0·35–0·5 micrograms kg^{-1} per minute, to improve renal, mesenteric, splanchnic, and hepatic blood flow, which is thought to be beneficial in preserving gastrointestinal mucosal integrity in certain patients. Dopexamine has been shown to improve outcome in certain high risk surgical patients (see Chapter 10). Like dopamine, there is no evidence to justify using dopexamine as a specific treatment for renal failure. The indications for and disadvantages of dopexamine are given in Box 6.5.

Box 6.5 Dopexamine indications and disadvantages

Indications
- Low cardiac output states
- Certain surgical patients

Disadvantages
- Tachycardia and arrythmias
- Myocardial ischaemia
- Nausea and vomiting
- Hypotension
- Angina
- Hypokalaemia and hypoglycaemia

Norepinephrine (noradrenaline)

Dose range is 0·01–0·4 micrograms kg^{-1} per minute. Norepinephrine is a potent α agonist (vasoconstrictor), raising blood pressure by increasing systemic vascular resistance. It has some $\beta1$ receptor activity causing increased contractility, heart rate, and cardiac output but it has no effect on $\beta2$ receptors. It increases myocardial oxygen demands without increasing coronary blood flow. It acts mainly as a vasopressor, with little inotropic effect. Norepinephrine reduces renal, hepatic, and muscle blood flow but, in patients with severe sepsis, it can increase renal blood flow and urine output by increasing perfusion pressure. The indications for and disadvantages of norepinephrine are given in Box 6.6.

Box 6.6 Norepinephrine (noradrenaline) indications and disadvantages

Indications
- Septic shock with low SVR
- Treatment of hypotension caused by vasodilation, e.g. regional anaesthesia

Disadvantages
- Excessive vasoconstriction
- Myocardial ischaemia
- Bradyarrhythmias and tachyarrhythmias

Table 6.3 Summary of inotrope actions

Inotropes	α	β1	β2	DA
Dobutamine		+++	++	
Adrenaline	+ to +++	+++	++	
Dopamine				
0–3 micrograms kg^{-1} per minute				+++
2·5–10 micrograms kg^{-1} per minute		++	+	++
> 10 micrograms kg^{-1} per minute	++	++	+	+
Dopexamine		+	+++	++
Noradrenaline	+++	+		

All these drugs are short-acting and their effects on the circulation are seen immediately (however, a CVP line has a 1 ml dead space capacity so there is a delay before onset of action unless the drug is bolused along the line first). They should be increased at frequent intervals (for example, every 15 minutes) until either the desired effect has occurred or an optimum dose has been reached. A summary of inotrope actions on different receptors is shown in Table 6.3.

Invasive monitoring in circulatory failure

The central venous pressure (CVP) catheter

Central venous cannulation is used for:

- delivering irritant or vasoactive drugs
- CVP measurement

- as a conduit for example, pacing wires
- venous access.

The CVP is expressed in mmHg when transduced (in which case a mean value is taken) or cm H_2O if measured by a manometer (in which case the value at end-expiration is used); 10 mmHg is equivalent to 13 cm H_2O. Errors in measurement are commonplace in areas where staff are not familiar with the equipment.

The CVP is diminished by reduced venous return, which is caused by hypovolaemia or vasodilatation. Both of these require volume replacement. However, several factors cause the CVP to rise:

- raised intrathoracic pressure, for example IPPV
- right heart failure
- lung diseases with pulmonary hypertension, for example COPD
- compensatory vasoconstriction in healthy people, for example bleeding
- tension pneumothorax, constrictive pericarditis, or tamponade.

The most important concept is that the CVP is a pressure not a volume. Many things affect the pressure in the right heart that have nothing to do with volume:

- valve disease
- lung disease (afterload)
- vasoconstriction or dilation (preload)
- muscle compliance
- atrial size.

So, although the CVP is being used as an estimate of left ventricular filling pressure, it has several limitations. Single readings cannot influence management. It is the response of the CVP to fluid challenges that can help to assess volume status – it is possible to have a high CVP and to be volume depleted.

As mentioned in the previous chapter, the "rule of threes" is useful guide to fluid therapy. Generally, if the CVP remains unchanged or rises but then falls back to the original value after 5 minutes, a further fluid challenge should be administered. If the CVP rises and remains elevated, no further fluid is indicated.

The pulmonary artery (PA) catheter

The PA catheter is an attempt to measure left heart function more directly than the CVP – but there are still many variables. It was introduced into clinical practice in the 1970s by Swan and Ganz. The balloon-tipped catheter is 70 cm long, with markings every 10 cm. The catheter has several channels including some for infusions, inflating the balloon, and connections to a thermistor. PA catheters enable therapy to be flow-based by measuring the following:

• right atrial, ventricular, and pulmonary artery occlusion pressures
• cardiac output/index
• derived data for systemic vascular resistance
• mixed venous O_2 saturation used to assess oxygen delivery and uptake.

Complications of the PA catheter (in addition to those of the CVP) include:

• arrhythmias (50%; sustained or clinically important arrhythmias are uncommon)
• catheter knotting
• damage to valves or myocardium (for example, mural thrombus 30–60%)
• pulmonary infarction (0·1–7%)
• pulmonary artery rupture (< 0·1%)
• the reliance on numbers rather than clinical assessment.

An introducer is inserted into the right internal jugular or left subclavian vein. After the catheter has been prepared, it is connected to a pressure transducer. The catheter is inserted to 20 cm, beyond the length of the introducer and in the large veins. The balloon is then inflated and the catheter inserted further. The balloon helps the catheter tip move with blood

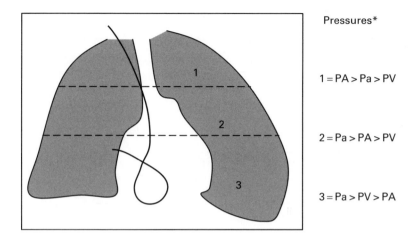

Pressures*

1 = PA > Pa > PV

2 = Pa > PA > PV

3 = Pa > PV > PA

Figure 6.2 PA catheter appearance on a chest x ray film. The PA catheter is still indirect. The catheter curls in the right ventricle and the tip sits in the pulmonary artery (lungs) but is trying to measure pressure changes in the left ventricle – via the whole of the lungs, left atrium, and mitral valve. The PA catheter tip must sit in a West zone 3 of the lung. West described physiological lung zones; zone 3 is where pulmonary venous pressure is greater than alveolar pressure. If the tip is in a non-zone 3, the wedge pressure may reflect alveolar rather than left atrial pressure. Luckily, balloon catheters tend to enter zone 3 because it is the area with highest blood flow. Although West zones are anatomical in normal lungs, they are actually physiological zones which can be altered by disease. Absence of a normal waveform, a wedge pressure that fluctuates widely with respiration or a rise in wedge pressure greater than half of any PEEP increase are clues to a non-zone 3 placement
*Pressure in the pulmonary arteries (Pa), alveolus (PA) and veins (PV).

flow to the right place (Figure 6.2) – hence the expression "floating a PA catheter".

When the catheter tip is wedged, it directly communicates with the left atrium via the pulmonary vessels (Figure 6.3). The pulmonary artery occlusion pressure (PAOP) is approximately the same as left atrial pressure. At end-diastole, left atrial pressure approximates to left ventricular pressure, which in turn is assumed to reflect left ventricular end-diastolic

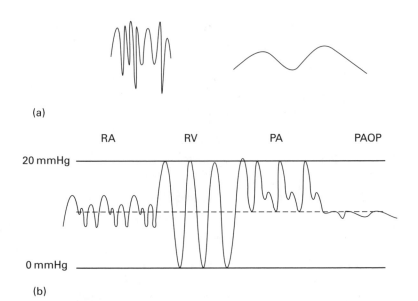

Figure 6.3 PA catheter trace patterns. (a) Waving the catheter tip in mid-air before insertion produces a trace like this. Air bubbles damp the trace as on the right hand side and should be flushed out. (b) First a characteristic central venous pressure (CVP) trace is seen, followed by a right ventricular (RV) trace as soon as the catheter tip enters the right ventricle (note the higher pressures). When the catheter tip enters the pulmonary artery (PA), the diastolic pressure increases and the trace changes to have a dichotic notch. When the balloon wedges, a damped trace is seen. The catheter must not be left wedged as pulmonary infarction may occur – this is for measurements only. In a healthy unventilated patient CVP = PAOP. PAOP, pulmonary artery occlusion pressure; RA, right atrium

volume. Readings are taken at end-expiration when intrathoracic pressure is nearest to zero. Lung and mitral valve disease are two major factors affecting the assumption that PAOP is equivalent to left ventricular end-diastolic volume. Pulmonary vascular resistance is increased in mitral stenosis, hypoxaemia, acidosis, pulmonary embolism, and acute respiratory distress syndrome (ARDS). A stiff left ventricle alters the relationship between pressure and volume. Furthermore, many values from the PA catheter are calculated

Table 6.4 Normal PA catheter values and intracardiac pressures

Value	Normal range
CVP	0–8 mmHg (aim for > 10 if starts low)
Right ventricle	0–8 mmHg diastolic, 15–30 mmHg systolic
PAOP	5–15 mmHg
Left atrium	4–12 mmHg
Left ventricle	4–12 mmHg diastolic, 90–140 mmHg systolic
Stroke volume	55–100 ml
CO	4–8 litres per minute
CI	1·5–4 litres per minute m^{-2}
SVR	770–1500 dyn.s cm^{-5}

CI, cardiac index; CO, cardiac output; CVP, central venous pressure; PAOP, pulmonary artery occlusion pressure; SVR, systemic vascular resistance.

from other measurements rather than measured directly, so entering the incorrect weight and height of the patient can also introduce error.

Again, trends are more important than a single reading and should be used in conjunction with a thorough clinical assessment. Clinical assessment still remains far more important than numbers alone. PA catheter values are shown in Table 6.4.

Cardiac output is measured by the thermodilution method. Cold fluid is injected rapidly via the proximal PA catheter lumen into the right atrium at end-expiration. The thermistor measures the temperature change downstream and a computer calculates CO using the indicator dilution equation.

PA catheters are indicated when there is an operator experienced in their use and the risk:benefit ratio to the patient is acceptable. Although practice varies, examples of PA catheter use are:

- to monitor the effects of therapy, for example in septic shock where more than one vasoactive drug may be required;
- in right-sided myocardial infarctions where right and left ventricular pressures are very different;
- to distinguish cardiogenic from non-cardiogenic pulmonary oedema in severe sepsis.

Mini-tutorial: controversy around the use of the PA catheter

There has been little evidence to show that the use of PA catheters improves outcome. Recently, a small number of papers were published which suggested that PA catheters actually caused harm. The paper by Connors *et al.* is one example. They looked at nearly 6000 patients going through an ICU in the USA. Just over 2000 had PA catheters. They adjusted for severity of illness and paired PA catheter patients with similar non-PA catheter patients. The PA catheter patients had worse outcomes and longer ICU stays (thus increasing costs). Possible explanations include:

• Clinicians tend to put PA catheters in patients who are sicker and not responding to conventional therapy.
• Clinicians may not be using the PA catheter appropriately – that is, relying on numbers rather than clinical assessment.
• Studies in the USA may not apply to European intensive care practice.

Several randomised controlled trials are now in progress to answer these questions and early results suggest that PA catheters do not increase mortality. Rhodes *et al.* looked at 200 patients in intensive care. In this study the PA catheter did not affect outcome either way. Clinicians were allowed to use clinical discretion when manipulating haemodynamic values rather than work to a protocol, and this fact may be significant. Larger trials are awaited that will help to answer the question of PA catheter use more definitively. In the meantime, use of PA catheters varies between different intensive care units.

Other ways to measure cardiac output

Because of the invasiveness of the PA catheter, people have looked to develop other ways of measuring cardiac output in the clinical setting. Whilst the PA catheter is considered the "gold standard", advances in computer technology, sensor design and refined interpretation of data have allowed the development of useful methods of measuring cardiac output without invasive vascular access. Transoesophageal echocardiography probes can estimate stroke volume. Doppler imaging can measure the velocity of blood in the ascending aorta. The length of a column of blood passing through the aorta in unit time can be measured. This is multiplied by the cross-sectional area of the aorta to give stroke volume. However, this is not feasible for continuous monitoring in awake patients. Thermodilution and pulse wave analysis techniques are also used. These more invasive techniques include the PiCCO (transpulmonary thermodilution and arterial pulse contour analysis), LIDCO (lithium dilution and arterial waveform analysis) and the Transonic (ultrasound indicator saline dilution) systems. The PiCCO system requires a central venous cannula and a thermistor-tipped femoral arterial line. The femoral arterial line allows pulse contour analysis and from this cardiac output is derived. A known volume of ice cold saline is rapidly injected into the central venous cannula. The injectate disperses into the lungs and all four cardiac chambers. A temperature difference reaches the femoral thermistor and a dissipation curve is generated. The global end-diastolic volume can be estimated from this and this reflects changes in volume status.

The NiCO system uses the indirect Fick principle using carbon dioxide rebreathing but requires intubation rather than vascular access.

Many of the advances in non-invasive cardiac output monitoring include the ability to monitor parameters continuously and to follow trends in therapy and interventions. The most impressive advance in non-invasive cardiac output monitoring has been the development of reliable techniques using advanced forms of thoracic bio-impedance measurements. The EIC (electrical impedance cardiography) and CBII (chest baseline impedance independent) systems are able to provide continuous trend monitoring of heart rate and stroke volume giving derived cardiac output and index parameters using stroke waveform morphology analysis.

The real advantage of these truly non-invasive techniques is the opportunity to begin monitoring these parameters in the Emergency Department, ward, or Coronary Care Unit before admission to the ICU becomes necessary or possible.

Pump failure

Cardiogenic shock can be split into two main categories: shock due to pump failure or shock due to mechanical complications of infarction (for example, acute valve failure, tamponade, or acute ventricular septal defects) which will not be discussed further. Over the last 20 years there have been major advances in the treatment of myocardial infarction and in outcome. Despite this the incidence and outcome from cardiogenic shock has remained roughly the same. It is a major cause of death among patients with acute coronary syndromes. The incidence of cardiogenic shock is around 7–10%. The majority occurs after ST elevation myocardial infarction, but 3% occurs in patients with unstable angina and 2% in patients with non-ST elevation MI. Hospital mortality is 45–80%.

Randomised trials have tended to define cardiogenic shock as a systolic blood pressure of < 90 mmHg for at least 1 hour that is not responsive to fluid administration alone, that is secondary to cardiac dysfunction, or that is associated with signs of hypoperfusion (or cardiac index < 2·2 litre per minute m^{-2} and pulmonary capillary wedge pressure more than 18 mmHg). In essence, the mainstay of diagnosis is a sustained systolic blood pressure of < 90 mmHg with evidence of organ hypoperfusion.

Principles in the management of cardiogenic shock

Cardiogenic shock has a high mortality. If hypoperfusion is present (see previous chapter), early intervention is required. A summary of the interventions in cardiogenic shock is given in Box 6.7.

Box 6.7 Interventions in cardiogenic shock

- Reversible causes of pump failure – correct mechanical problems, heart rate, hypoxaemia, drug effects and hypocalcaemia
- Reversible ischaemia – thrombolysis is a priority if indicated. Anti platelet agents should be given. Other interventions may be indicated as directed by a cardiologist
- Suboptimal preload – assess volume status using fluid challenges and achieve effective circulating volume
- Haemodynamic data required – CVP line, urinary catheter, arterial line, (cardiac output measurements)
- Low cardiac output despite optimum heart rate and filling pressures – start dobutamine. If hypoperfusion still present at optimum doses, add a drug with α effects. Intra-aortic balloon pumping may also be used

---

Identify and treat patients in the preshock state early and effectively instead of waiting to take action once shock is established. When acidosis from hypoperfusion occurs, myocardial function is further depressed, vasoactive drugs are less likely to work, and it may be difficult to break the physiological downward spiral. Patients treated early but who fail to respond to optimum therapy are unlikely to have any significant cardiac reserve and have a poor prognosis.

Clinical assessment of a patient with circulatory failure

A and B are still important in a patient with circulatory failure. This is because the reason the circulation exists is to get oxygen to the cells. Airway and breathing play a vital role in this function. After that, circulation can be optimised. The use of inotropes nearly always follows the use of fluid and there is a constant cycle of re-assessment (Figure 6.4).

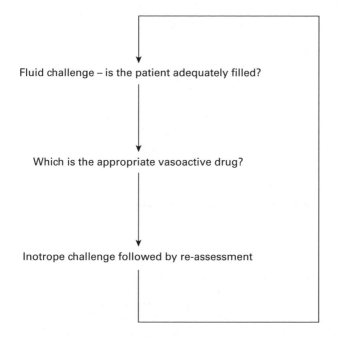

Fluid challenge – is the patient adequately filled?

Which is the appropriate vasoactive drug?

Inotrope challenge followed by re-assessment

Figure 6.4 Cycle of re-assessment in circulatory failure

The best inotrope or inotrope combination will vary not only between patients with the same condition but also in the same patient over the course of their illness. If there is no satisfactory response to an optimum dose of one inotrope, a different drug should be considered. Remember the things which affect cardiac output or flow:

$$CO = HR \times SV \text{ (contractility/inotropy, preload, afterload)}$$

and the things which affect blood pressure:

$$BP = CO \times SVR$$

All of these variables should be considered and manipulated to get the best organ perfusion possible.

Self-assessment – case histories

1. A 50-year-old man is admitted with an anterior myocardial infarction and develops hypotension 12 hours later with a poor urine output. His vital signs are: pulse 90 per minute, blood pressure 80/50 mmHg, respiratory rate 20 per minute, SaO_2 95% on air, temperature 37°C and he is alert. What is your management?

2. A 60-year-old man is admitted to the HDU for "pre-optimisation" 12 hours before a laparotomy. He is treated normally for hypertensive heart failure and this is controlled. He has developed sepsis. He has warm, dry peripheries and his vital signs are: pulse 98 per minute, blood pressure 110/70 mmHg, respiratory rate 26 per minute, SaO_2 96% on air, temperature 37·5°C and he is alert. He says he is thirsty. His PA catheter readings are as follows:

    - CVP = 14 mmHg
    - PAOP = 10 (8–12 mmHg)
    - CO = 5·5 (4–8 litres per minute), CI = 3 (1·5–4 litres per minute m^{-2})
    - SVR = 1100 (770–1500 dyn.s cm^{-5})

    How would you optimise this patient?

3. A 40-year-old man is admitted with a severe gastrointestinal bleed. His vital signs are: pulse 100 per minute, blood pressure 150/70 mmHg, respiratory rate 20 per minute, SaO_2 98% on air; he is alert and has cold hands and feet. A CVP line is inserted. The first reading is 16 mmHg. The doctor decides not to give

further fluid and observe the patient. What would your management plan be?

4. You are called to see a postoperative patient who has developed a poor urine output (< 0·5 mg kg^{-1} per hour for 2 consecutive hours). His vital signs are: pulse 90 per minute, blood pressure 120/70 mmHg, respiratory rate 20 per minute, SaO_2 95% on 2 litres per minute oxygen via nasal cannulae. His chest is clear. His arterial blood gases show: pH 7·34, $PaCO_2$ 4·0 kPa (30·7 mmHg), PaO_2 10·0 kPa (77 mmHg) and bicarbonate 13 mmol/l, BE − 8. His CVP reading is 12 mmHg. He has mild peripheral oedema. What would your management plan be?

5. A patient is admitted with an inferior myocardial infarction. His pulse is 40 per minute (sinus bradycardia) and blood pressure 95/60 mmHg. His urine output is satisfactory. His hands are warm, his respiratory rate is 16 per minute, temperature 36·5°C and SaO_2 96% on air. What is your management?

6. You are asked to see an 80-year-old lady because she has a low blood pressure. On examination her vital signs are: pulse 70 per minute, blood pressure 90/60 mmHg, respiratory rate 14 per minute, SaO_2 95% on air. She has warm hands and feet and is mobile on the ward. What other parameters would you assess and what is your management?

7. A patient has developed low blood pressure on the coronary care unit. One examination the vital signs are: pulse 180 per minute, blood pressure 80/50 mmHg, respiratory rate 18 per minute, SaO_2 80% on air. He has cold hands. What is the cause of the low oxygen saturations and what is your management?

8. A 40-year-old man is admitted to ICU with hypotension causing hypoperfusion that has not responded to fluid challenges. He has a PA catheter inserted and the initial readings show:

- CVP = 3 mmHg
- PAOP = 5 (8–12 mmHg)
- CO = 10 (4–8 litres per minute), CI = 4·5 (1·5–4 litres per minute m^{-2})
- SVR = 300 (770–1500 dyn.s cm^{-5})

What diagnosis are these readings consistent with? What would your management be?

Self-assessment − discussion

1. Immediate management includes the following: airway and breathing should be assessed and treated before circulation. The hypotension is causing renal hypoperfusion and should be treated without delay. When any mechanical causes for cardiac failure has been excluded, the response to a fluid challenge should be assessed. When preload has been optimised, it would be appropriate to start an inotrope and assess the

response to this. Intra-aortic balloon pumping should be considered. Further fluid challenges and other vasoactive drugs may be required.

2. Airway and breathing should be assessed and treated first. Ignore the PA catheter readings and assess the patient clinically. What is his normal blood pressure? Are there signs of hypoperfusion (What is the urine output and base excess)? He has warm, dry skin, is tachycardic, and says he is thirsty. He has a history consistent with volume depletion – sepsis and perhaps chronic diuretic use. A fluid challenge is indicated. In a patient with sepsis, one would expect to find a raised cardiac output and a low SVR. This patient's response has been altered by heart failure, so although these readings appear "normal", they do not indicate normal physiology.

3. After A and B, circulation is assessed by looking at the vital signs and for signs of hypoperfusion (for example, skin temperature). This patient has cold peripheries and is tachycardic. A 40-year-old man with a severe GI bleed may compensate by vasoconstriction and this raises the CVP. Single CVP readings are rarely useful. His volume status should be assessed with fluid challenges and the response of his vital signs and CVP readings to these.

4. A and B should be assessed and treated first. In terms of circulation, he has a "normal" blood pressure, but there are signs of hypoperfusion – poor urine output and a metabolic acidosis. The response of the urine output, base deficit, and CVP to fluid challenges should be assessed.

5. This patient is hypotensive but not hypoperfused. He is exhibiting the Bezold–Jarisch reflex – a response of coronary artery chemoreceptors to ischaemia causing hypotension and bradycardia. This is designed to increased coronary blood flow. Any poor urine output that occurs normally responds to a fluid challenge.

6. This patient is hypotensive but not hypoperfused. What is her normal blood pressure? No emergency intervention is indicated.

7. Airway and breathing should be assessed and treated. If the patient is alert and talking, the airway is secure. A high concentration of oxygen should be given (for example, 15 litres per minute via a simple face mask or reservoir bag mask). Assessment of the circulation reveals a low blood pressure causing hypoperfusion. His heart rate is 180 per minute and this should be treated first (Figure 6.5). In a compromised patient, DC cardioversion is indicated. A return to sinus rhythm will probably restore perfusion. His low oxygen saturations are probably caused by a weak signal from hypoperfusion and tachycardia rather than hypoxaemia – arterial blood gas analysis will confirm this.

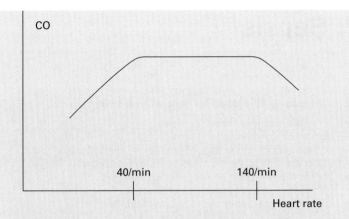

Figure 6.5 The Treppe effect of heart rate on cardiac output (CO) (*treppe* means staircase)

8. These readings show low filling pressures (low CVP and PAOP), high cardiac output, and low systemic vascular resistance. This is consistent with a diagnosis of severe sepsis. Fluid challenges should be given to optimise filling pressures. A persistently low SVR despite this is treated with vasopressors.

Further reading

Connors AF, Speroff T, Dawson NV *et al.* The effectiveness of right heart catheterisation in the initial care or critically ill patients. SUPPORT Investigators. *JAMA* 1996;**276**:889–97.

Lin ES, Duthie DR. Physiology of the circulation. In: Pinnock C, Lin T, Smith T, eds. *Fundamentals of Anaesthesia*. London: Medical Media Ltd, 1999.

Manikon M, Grounds M, Rhodes A. The pulmonary artery catheter. *Clin Med* 2002;**2**:101–4.

Rhodes A, Cusack RJ, Newman PJ, Grounds RM, Bennet ED. A randomised controlled trial of the pulmonary artery catheter in critically ill patients. *Intens Care Med* 2002;**28**:256–64.

Swanevelder JLC. Cardiac physiology. In: Pinnock C, Lin T, Smith T, eds. *Fundamentals of Anaesthesia*. London, Medical Media Ltd, 1999.

Williams SG, Wright DJ, Tan L-B. Management of cardiogenic shock complicating acute myocardial infarction: towards evidence based medical practice. *Heart* 2000;**83**:621–6.

7: Sepsis

By the end of this chapter you will be able to:

- be aware of the terminology used
- understand the underlying pathophysiology of sepsis
- understand the principles of circulatory resuscitation in sepsis
- understand the role of intensive care in supporting patients
- appreciate the effects of sepsis on the lung
- be aware of recent advances in therapy
- know about microbiological considerations
- apply this to your clinical practice

The incidence of sepsis is increasing and is a major cause of morbidity and mortality in hospital. It is the leading cause of death in UK ICUs. The increasing use of immunosuppressant agents, broad-spectrum antibiotics, and invasive technology is contributing to the rising incidence. Around one-third of UK ICU admissions are now due to severe sepsis. In the USA the annual incidence of sepsis is in the order of 400 000 per year with 200 000 cases of septic shock and an estimated 100 000 deaths. In Holland it has been recorded that severe sepsis occurs in 13·6 per 1000 and septic shock in 4·6 per 100 hospital admissions. Early recognition and treatment is vital – once organ failure is established, mortality is over 50% (Table 7.1).

Terminology

In 1991 a consensus conference produced definitions of sepsis and its adverse sequelae. The term systemic inflammatory

Table 7.1 Mortality rates in the sepsis continuum (mortality also increases with age)

Diagnosis	Mortality (%)
Bacteraemia	10–20
Bacteraemia + sepsis	20–30
Severe sepsis	40–60
Sepsis + multiple organ failure	over 80

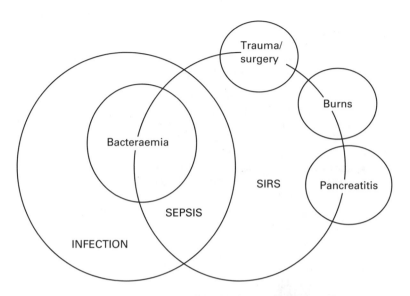

Figure 7.1 Systemic inflammatory response syndrome and sepsis

response syndrome (SIRS) defines the clinical manifestations of the widespread inflammation that results from a variety of insults including infection, pancreatitis, burns, and trauma including surgery (Figure 7.1). Sepsis is defined as the systemic inflammatory response to a documented infection. Severe sepsis is associated with organ dysfunction and hypoperfusion. Septic shock refers to those patients who remain hypotensive despite adequate fluid resuscitation. Box 7.1 shows the definitions in the sepsis continuum.

The term multiple organ dysfunction syndrome (MODS) is a clinical syndrome in which the development of progressive and potentially reversible physiological dysfunction in two or more organ systems occurs. It is induced by a variety of acute insults and its occurrence in sepsis is characteristic. MODS is a continuum – varying from a mild degree of dysfunction to frank organ failure.

Pathophysiology of sepsis

The features seen in sepsis are the result of an inflammatory response to a invading organism. This involves the production

Box 7.1 Definitions in the sepsis continuum

- Infection – invasion of micro-organisms into a normally sterile site, often associated with an inflammatory host response
- Bacteraemia – viable bacteria in the blood stream
- Septicaemia – no uniform definition, often interpreted as bacteraemia plus severe illness
- Sepsis – clinical evidence of infection plus a systemic response indicated by two or more of the following:
  - hyper (> 38°C) or hypothermia (< 36°C)
  - tachycardia (heart rate > 90/minute)
  - tachypnoea (respiratory rate > 20/minute)
  - white blood cells > 12×10^9 or < 4×10^9 or "left shift"
- Severe sepsis – sepsis associated with organ dysfunction:
  - hypotension
  - poor urine output
  - hypoxaemia
  - confusion
  - metabolic acidosis
  - disseminated intravascular coagulation
- Septic shock – severe sepsis with hypotension unresponsive to intravascular volume replacement
- Refractory shock – hypotension not responding to vasoactive drugs

of cytokines, nitric oxide, thromboxanes, leukotrienes, platelet activating factor, prostaglandins, and complement. There is also activation of coagulation and platelet aggregation. All this leads to:

- increased capillary permeability
- hypovolaemia, hypoperfusion, and a disturbed microcirculation
- development of a metabolic acidosis with increasing blood lactate
- impaired oxygen utilisation
- reduced myocardial contractility caused by circulating myocardial depressants, acidosis, and hypoxaemia
- a reduced systemic vascular resistance (SVR)
- increased pulmonary vascular resistance
- increased oxygen extraction owing to a hypermetabolic state
- coagulopathy with microvascular thrombosis.

The "typical" patient with severe sepsis has a fever and tachycardia, and is vasodilated with an increased cardiac output and low blood pressure. However, poor myocardial function is also part of severe sepsis and may contribute to hypotension. Patients can appear vasoconstricted with cold peripheries especially if there is coexisting hypovolaemia. It is important to recognise that sepsis is a dynamic process with rapid evolution of physical signs covering a wide continuum of physiological responses.

The host response to infection is protective – but in severe sepsis it seems to be stimulated excessively leading to organ dysfunction, multiple organ failure, and death. In simplified terms, severe sepsis can be thought of as dysfunction between the opposing mechanisms that normally maintain homeostasis. The main systems that become dysfunctional in severe sepsis are inflammation, coagulation/fibrinolysis, and the endothelium. Other factors such as mitochondrial dysfunction also play a role.

Inflammation

The body's initial response to a pro-inflammatory insult is to release mediators like tumour necrosis factor (TNF), interleukin 1, interleukin 6, and platelet-activating factor (PAF). These mediators have multiple overlapping effects designed to repair existing damage and limit new damage. To ensure that the effects of the pro-inflammatory mediators do not become destructive, the body then launches compensatory anti-inflammatory mediators like interleukin 4 and interleukin 10, which downregulate the initial pro-inflammatory response. In severe sepsis, regulation of the early response to a pro-inflammatory insult is lost and a massive systemic reaction occurs with excessive or inappropriate inflammatory reactions, resulting in the development of diffuse capillary injury.

Coagulation

As well as inflammation, there are abnormalities of both coagulation (clot formation) and fibrinolysis (break down of clot) as illustrated in Figure 7.2.

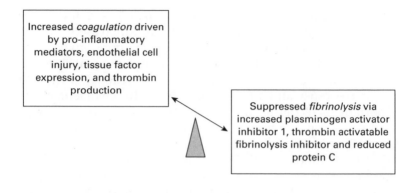

Increased *coagulation* driven by pro-inflammatory mediators, endothelial cell injury, tissue factor expression, and thrombin production

Suppressed *fibrinolysis* via increased plasminogen activator inhibitor 1, thrombin activatable fibrinolysis inhibitor and reduced protein C

Figure 7.2 Abnormalities of coagulation and fibrinolysis

The many inflammatory mediators that are released promote coagulation. In addition, infectious agents can cause endothelial damage themselves, which also promotes coagulation. At each step in the cycle auto-amplification occurs, accelerating the coagulation abnormalities. Pro-inflammatory cytokines, such as interleukin 1A, interleukin 1B, and TNF, induce the expression of tissue factor (TF) on endothelial cells and monocytes initiating coagulation. TF is a key mediator between the immune system and coagulation and is the principle activator of coagulation causing large amounts of thrombin to be generated.

Fibrinolysis

The end result of the clotting pathway is the production of thrombin, which converts soluble fibrinogen to insoluble fibrin. The fibrin aggregates and forms a clot together with platelets, blocking the damaged blood vessel and preventing further bleeding. The fibrinolytic system (Figure 7.3) is directly influenced by the septic process and, in most patients with sepsis, it is suppressed while coagulation proceeds. Two key inhibitors of fibrinolysis that are produced by sepsis are plasminogen activator inhibitor 1 and thrombin activeatable fibrinolysis inhibitor.

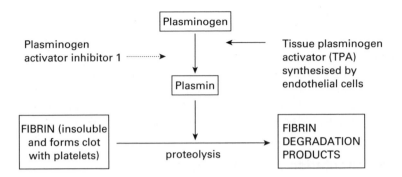

Figure 7.3 Fibrinolysis (clot breakdown). Venous occlusion or thrombin stimulates tissue plasminogen activator release. Sepsis produces PAI –1. Activated protein C inactivates PAI –1. Fibrin degradation products (FDPs) are used clinically to measure the activity of the fibrinolytic system, but d-dimers are more specific – produced by the digestion of cross-linked fibrin

Bleeding

Coagulation and fibrinolysis are usually finely balanced. Inappropriate activation of the coagulation cascade results in widespread fibrin deposition (clot formation), and coagulation factors and platelets are consumed faster than they can be replaced. Hence the paradox of both microvascular thrombosis and bleeding. The fibrin strands fragment passing red blood cells and the resulting microangiopathic haemolysis may be seen on the blood film.

The following laboratory changes are therefore seen in severe sepsis:

- reduced platelets
- prolonged APTT, PT, and TT
- reduced fibrinogen
- elevated d-dimer
- microangiopathic haemolysis leading to anaemia and reticulocytosis.

This picture is described as disseminated intravascular coagulation (DIC).

The endothelium

The normal role of the endothelium includes interaction with leucocytes, the release of cytokines and inflammatory mediators, the release of mediators of vasodilatation and vasoconstriction, and a part in the coagulation system. In severe sepsis there is physical as well as chemical dysfunction of the endothelium. Holes appear, which lead to persistent capillary leak.

The circulation in severe sepsis

There is a common failure to understand that the hypovolaemia in patients with severe sepsis requires successive fluid challenges rather than a simple fluid infusion. Large fluid deficits can result from diarrhoea or third space losses in peritonitis, but vasodilatation and capillary leak also lead to dramatic intravascular volume depletion. Fluid challenges should be titrated to the clinical endpoints of blood pressure, heart rate, urine output, and other markers of perfusion. In persistent hypotension with hypoperfusion, it is essential that the attending doctor stays with the patient until acceptable parameters have been reached or the patient is transferred to the ICU for further monitoring and treatment with vasoactive drugs.

Invasive or more sophisticated monitoring than simple pulse, blood pressure, and urine output should be instituted early in severe sepsis. Early goal-directed therapy has been shown to improve outcome. Severe sepsis is a complex ICU disease. Close attention must be paid during the administration of fluids as signs of pulmonary oedema and bilateral infiltrates on the chest *x* ray film can appear without obvious fluid overload if ARDS is present (see later). PA catheters are often used in severe sepsis precisely because it can be difficult to evaluate the degree of hypovolaemia, the presence of cardiac dysfunction, and thus the aetiology of any pulmonary oedema.

Unlike other causes of shock, the cardiac output is often maintained or even increased in severe sepsis. Septic shock results from alterations in the distribution of blood flow. There is loss of control of the microvasculature with the abnormal distribution of cardiac output. Reduced oxygen and nutrient delivery to the tissues causes organ dysfunction. The goal of therapy is therefore to restore tissue perfusion through the use of fluids and vasoactive drugs.

Systemic vascular resistance (SVR) can be measured by invasive and non-invasive means and is of great value in titrating vasoactive drugs in severe sepsis, when the SVR is usually low. SVR may be thought of as the resistance against which the heart pumps. It is calculated using a PA catheter as follows:

$$\text{SVR in dyn.s cm}^{-5} = \frac{\text{MAP} - \text{CVP in mmHg} \times 80 \text{ (correction factor)}}{\text{CO in litres per minute}}$$

The normal range is 1000–1500 dyn.s cm^{-5}. SVR is mainly determined by the diameter of arterioles, which is affected by intrinsic autoregulation, locally produced substances that vasodilate (for example, nitric oxide), hypoxaemia, neural factors, and circulating toxins. SVR increases with normal ageing in Western populations. SVR $\times$ body surface area in kg m^{-2} gives the systemic vascular resistance index (SVRI), which is often used in clinical practice.

Ideally, blood pressure is measured invasively with an arterial line, as measurement of blood pressure with a cuff is often unreliable and inaccurate at low blood pressures. The level of mean arterial pressure (MAP) to aim for is not clear but most studies have shown that a MAP of < 60 mmHg is associated with compromised autoregulation in the coronary, renal, and brain circulations. MAP is not commonly used on general wards – a practical guide is that you should aim for a blood pressure that adequately perfuses the tissues and this is usually – but not always – > 90 mmHg systolic. To a certain extent adequate perfusion depends on the patient's usual blood pressure, which should be identified if possible. Some patients require higher pressures for adequate perfusion.

Mini-tutorial: dopamine or norepinephrine (noradrenaline) in septic shock?

Dopamine

Clinicians vary in the use of high dose dopamine or norepinephrine in septic shock. There are several theoretical reasons why norepinephrine is better and this is supported by some studies. Much of our knowledge of the effects of dopamine comes from healthy humans. Dopamine is a naturally occurring catecholamine. You may recall that dopaminergic receptor stimulation predominates at low doses, causing an increase in renal and mesenteric flow. β1 stimulation occurs at moderate doses causing increased myocardial contractility, heart rate, and cardiac output; α stimulation occurs at higher doses, increasing systemic vascular resistance and reducing renal blood flow. In the critically ill, there is wide interpatient variation in plasma clearance of dopamine. In healthy humans, dopamine infusions have theoretical beneficial effects on renal and splanchnic circulations but this has not translated into improved outcomes in studies. In fact, there is some evidence to suggest that dopamine may have detrimental effects on the splanchnic circulation in patients with sepsis.

Norepinephrine (noradrenaline)

Septic shock is characterised by a high cardiac output, low systemic vascular resistance, and a normal or low pulmonary arterial occlusion pressure. Norepinephrine is a potent α receptor agonist, that is, it vasoconstricts. It also stimulates β1 receptors at higher doses, increasing cardiac output, but has no effect on β2 receptors. If norepinephrine is used in patients with uncorrected hypovolaemia, or in haemorrhagic shock, it has severe detrimental effects on tissue perfusion, particularly in the kidneys. Norepinephrine reduces renal, hepatic, and muscle blood flow but, when used in patients with septic shock who have been adequately fluid resuscitated, norepinephrine improves both urine production and renal function. This is because it improves renal perfusion pressure by raising blood pressure.

One prospective, double-blind, randomised trial compared norepinephrine and dopamine in the treatment of septic shock. Patients with similar characteristics were assigned to receive either norepinephrine 0·5–5 micrograms kg^{-1} per minute or dopamine 2·5–25 micrograms kg^{-1} per minute. If the haemodynamic and metabolic abnormalities were not corrected with the maximum dose of one drug then the other was added. The aim of therapy was to achieve for at least 6 hours an SVRI of > 1100 dyn.s cm^{-5} and/or a MAP of > 80 mmHg, a target cardiac index of > 4 litres per minute m^{-2} and normalisation of oxygen delivery and uptake. Only 31% patients were successfully treated with dopamine compared with 93% with norepinephrine. Ten of the 11 patients who did not respond to dopamine and remained hypotensive and oliguric were successfully treated with norepinephrine. The authors conclude that norepinephrine was more effective and reliable than dopamine in reversing the abnormalities in septic shock (defined by hypotension despite adequate fluid therapy with a low SVR, high cardiac output, oliguria, and lactic acidosis). A decrease in lactate levels was also seen with norepinephrine. The effects of norepinephrine on oxygen transport remain unclear from available data; however, most studies have found clinical parameters of peripheral perfusion to be significantly improved. Increased splanchnic blood flow has been demonstrated in patients with septic shock treated with norepinephrine.

Other inotropes used in septic shock

Dobutamine

Dobutamine is considered by many to be the pharmacological agent of choice to increase cardiac output when this is depressed in septic shock. It has a predominantly β1 effect that increases heart rate and contractility, hence cardiac output. It has no specific effects on renal blood flow but the increase in cardiac output can improve glomerular filtration rate.

Epinephrine (adrenaline)

In patients who have failed to respond to fluid administration or vasopressors, epinephrine can increase arterial pressure by increasing cardiac output and systemic vascular resistance.

Refractory shock

The role of steroids

The evidence for the use of steroids in the treatment of severe sepsis has gone full circle in the last 20 years, with recent interest focusing on low doses. In patients with severe sepsis there are complex effects on the hypothalamic–pituitary–adrenal axis. On the one hand there is stimulation of the axis and loss of negative feedback control, which usually leads to high adrenocorticotrope hormone (ACTH) and cortisol levels. On the other hand various mediators cause adrenal suppression and glucocorticoid resistance. With time ACTH levels may fall due to inhibition or pituitary depletion – this leads to relative adrenal suppression. Recent studies have shown that patients with sepsis who are dependent on vasoactive drugs may benefit from stress doses of hydrocortisone (50–100 mg intravenously 4 times a day for 7 days). A proportion of these have relative adrenal insufficiency as defined by the short synacthen test and these patients have the greatest benefit in terms of mortality. Whilst a proportion of patients may benefit, steroids are not a routine treatment in sepsis.

Plasmapheresis

Plasmapheresis is a non-selective method of removing toxic mediators from the circulation. Several reports have been published on the use of plasmapheresis in severe sepsis but these have been inconclusive. Plasma is removed from the circulation and replaced with donor fresh frozen plasma during plasmapheresis. The first prospective randomised controlled trial of plasmapheresis in septic shock has come from a Russian–Norwegian collaboration. They looked at 106 consecutive patients with severe sepsis or septic shock and randomised them to receive either standard therapy or add-on treatment with plasmapheresis. The patients had equivalent APACHE III scores at entry. The main endpoint was 28-day mortality: 33·3% (18/54) patients in the plasmapheresis group died compared with 53·8% (28/52) in the control group. This represented an absolute risk reduction of 20·5% with plasmapheresis. The number needed to treat was 4·9 patients with severe sepsis to prevent one death. Plasmapheresis appeared to be a safe procedure. However, the study population was heterogeneous with respect to the cause of sepsis. The authors concluded that a large multicentre prospective randomised controlled trial is needed to confirm these positive results.

Plasmapheresis lowers circulating endotoxins and cytokines, but replacement of donor plasma may also replenish deficiencies in immunoglobulins and clotting factors. There are immunological similarities between severe sepsis and thrombotic thrombocytopenic purpura (TTP) in which endothelial injury results in the release of multiple mediators and the presence of a large von Willebrand factor fragment. Plasmapheresis has lowered mortality in this condition from 90 to 10%. Patient selection may be important when using plasmapheresis in severe sepsis – but data on this are awaited. At the moment plasmapheresis is sometimes considered in patients with septic shock who are not responding to conventional therapy on the ICU.

Vasopressin

Endogenous vasopressin levels appear to be inappropriately low in severe sepsis compared with the raised levels seen in other shock states (for example, hypovolaemic and cardiogenic). Continuous infusion of vasopressin has been shown to have an effective pressor action in many patients with refractory shock, which is unresponsive to fluid resuscitation and noradrenaline. However, rebound hypotension often occurs on discontinuation of the drug.

Methylene blue

Methylene blue can be useful in elevating blood pressure in refractory shock with a bolus dose of 2 mg kg^{-1} over 15 minutes. It acts by inhibiting guanylate cyclase. Nitric oxide is formed from L-arginine by nitric oxide synthases. Nitric oxide stimulates guanylate cyclase to produce vasodilatation and reduced responsiveness to catecholamines. Methylene blue thus increases vascular tone.

Other supportive therapies

As sepsis is associated with multiple system organ failure, there are other supportive therapies used to treat these patients, which do not directly relate to the sepsis itself. Deep vein thrombosis (DVT) prophylaxis, nutritional support, and stress peptic ulcer prophylaxis are important adjuvant therapies. Nutritional support, especially enteral (via nasogastric tube) is important in supporting the hypercatabolic critically ill patient, preventing stress ulcers, and maintaining gut mucosal integrity. Tight glucose has also been shown to improve outcome.

Principles of resuscitation in severe sepsis

Hypoperfusion rapidly leads to organ dysfunction in severe sepsis. This systemic response to inflammation is an emergency. Immediate resuscitation should not be delayed by investigations as resuscitation can prevent further organ damage. A, B, C is more urgent than an exact diagnosis in the first instance. Diagnosis and the hunt for a source of infection can safely follow later. From the pathophysiology discussed so far, a methodical approach to resuscitation in severe sepsis is outlined in Box 7.2.

Box 7.2 Methodical approach to resuscitation in severe sepsis

A
- Reduced conscious level may compromise airway
- Oxygen therapy is needed

B
- Hypoperfusion and hypoxaemia increase the respiratory rate
- ARDS may be present
- Pneumonia can be the cause of severe sepsis

C
- Hypovolaemia requires successive fluid challenges
- Vasopressors may be needed because of an abnormally low SVR
- Reduced myocardial contractility may also require treatment
- Clotting abnormalities need correcting

D and E
- Arterial blood gases to assess A, B, and C
- Full examination is required to locate the source of inflammation, including microbiological screening and imaging

---

The role of intensive care in supporting patients with severe sepsis

The use of vasoactive drugs in severe sepsis should only follow adequate fluid resuscitation and this usually requires more extensive monitoring than can be done in an ordinary ward. In the ICU, therapeutic strategies are aimed at normalising as far as possible the global, regional, and microcirculatory defects in oxygen transport that occur in severe sepsis. These strategies are guided by the more explicit measurements of cardiac output and SVR. The effects of different vasoactive drugs on the microcirculation are also considered. Intubation and ventilation is an important part of the strategy to improve oxygen delivery (DO_2) and reduce uptake ($\dot{V}O_2$). Early referral to ICU should be considered in all patients with severe sepsis.

The lung in sepsis

The development of respiratory dysfunction in patients with sepsis lies on a continuum from subclinical disease to overwhelming organ dysfunction. At the worst end is the acute respiratory distress syndrome (ARDS), a severe form of acute lung injury (ALI). The definition of ARDS is adapted from the American European Consensus Conference held in 1994:

- acute in timing
- PaO_2 in mmHg/FIO_2 (for example, 0·6 for 60% oxygen) of ≤ 200
- bilateral infiltrates on the chest x ray film
- a pulmonary arterial occlusion pressure of < 18 mmHg.

These criteria show an incidence varying from 5 to 71 per 100 000 people in the USA and accounting for nearly 5 billion dollars' worth of financial support. Morbidity and mortality associated with ALI and ARDS is in excess of 40%. Mortality is often due to unresolved sepsis or multiple organ failure as opposed to progressive respiratory failure. The hallmark of ARDS is alveolar epithelial inflammation, air space flooding with plasma proteins and cellular debris, surfactant depletion and inactivation, and loss of normal endothelial reactivity.

Hypoxaemia in sepsis is caused by extensive right-to-left intrapulmonary shunting of blood, which may account for more than 25% of the total cardiac output (see Figure 4.2). Usually compensation occurs through hypoxaemic vasoconstriction, limiting the amount of shunt by reducing perfusion to poorly ventilated lung units. However, in states of lung injury, hypoxaemic vasoconstriction may be ineffective or even absent. The shunting of blood through non-ventilated lung units accounts for the relative refractory nature of hypoxaemia in ARDS. The hypoxaemia is often out of proportion to initial x ray film findings. Lung compliance is the change in volume for a given change in pressure and is reduced in ARDS because of small airway and alveolar collapse. In early ARDS the volume of functional lung is also reduced by alveolar oedema and surfactant abnormalities. There is also an increase in airway resistance caused by airway secretions, oedema, and mediators that provoke bronchospasm.

As a result of changes in lung compliance in ARDS, greater airway pressures are needed to achieve a given tidal volume. This increases the work of breathing, which is exacerbated by the increased respiratory rate seen in severe sepsis. Hypoxaemia in sepsis therefore results from the following:

- ventilation–perfusion mismatch
- respiratory muscle dysfunction
- decreased thoracic compliance
- increased airway resistance due to bronchoconstriction.

Oxygen delivery is also affected by upper airway obstruction where there is a reduced conscious level, circulatory collapse, metabolic acidosis, and reduced haemoglobin levels.

The pathological changes in ARDS are divided into three phases:

1. the early exudative phase (days 1–5), characterised by oedema and haemorrhage;
2. the fibroproliferative phase (days 6–10), characterised by organisation and repair;
3. the fibrotic phase (after 10 days) characterised by fibrosis.

These times are approximate and characteristic features in each phase often overlap. When the initial signs and symptoms of sepsis first appear, between 28–33% of patients meet the criteria for ARDS.

Since ARDS was first reported, mortality has remained relatively constant at 60–70%. More recent reports suggest that mortality has declined to around 40%. The explanation for this apparent improvement in patient outcome is not clear but could be due to differences in patient populations, changes in ventilation strategies, greater attention to fluid management, improved haemodynamic and nutritional support, improved antibiotics for hospital-acquired infections, or corticosteroid use (small randomised trials have suggested benefit with intravenous corticosteroid therapy in patients with a prolonged fibroproliferative phase of ARDS). No one therapeutic intervention has been proved to be effective in reducing the incidence of respiratory failure in sepsis nor its mortality.

Intubation and mechanical ventilation is considered early in severe sepsis, especially if ARDS is present. The indications for intubation include:

- patient cannot protect own airway;
- correction of refractory hypoxaemia – PaO_2 < 8·0 kPA (60 mmHg) – despite maximum oxygen therapy;
- respiratory rate > 35 per minute and vital capacity < 15 ml kg^{-1} – invasive ventilation alleviates the increased work of breathing allowing blood to be redirected to other vital organs.

Non-invasive ventilation has not been shown to be effective in ARDS, although limited data exist.

Much has been written on the different ventilatory strategies in ARDS, which is beyond the scope of this book. Pressure-controlled inverse ratio ventilation is often used as a means of recruiting non-ventilated lung units. Smaller tidal volumes limit barotrauma and volutrauma. Permissive hypercapnia means that the CO_2 is allowed to rise to allow these ventilation strategies. Prone positioning of the patient can improve oxygenation but has not been shown to improve outcome. Finally, fluid balance can be difficult in ARDS because overhydration can be a disadvantage when the lung has leaky capillaries – but cardiac function and organ perfusion also have to be optimised.

Recent advances in severe sepsis

In recent years many new therapies for sepsis have been tested in randomised trials. All have attempted to counteract the effects of sepsis mediators with the use of specific antibodies, inhibitors, or antagonists. These trials have tended not to have an effect on mortality. The most promising of new treatments is Drotrecogin Alfa (activated), a recombinant form of activated protein C.

Activated protein C

Drotrecogin Alfa (activated) is the first therapeutic intervention shown to reduce all-cause mortality in severe sepsis. At 28 days 24·7% of Drotrecogin Alfa (activated) patients died versus 30·8% of patients treated with placebo. There was a 19·4% reduction in the relative risk of death (numbers needed to treat = 16). Significant decreases in levels of protein C have been well documented in severe sepsis. The benefit of giving activated protein C is explained by the fact that it inhibits the generation of thrombin via inactivation of factor Va and VIIIa. D-dimer levels are seen to decrease in the first week of infusion and rise when the infusion is stopped. Activated protein C (APC) also reduces inflammation – interleukin 6 levels are reduced in studies. It is postulated that APC inhibits neutrophil activation, cytokine release, and adhesion of cells to the vascular endothelium, and has antithrombotic activity. Reductions in risk of death were seen whether or not patients had baseline low levels of activated protein C. Bleeding was the most common adverse event – one serious bleed occurred for every 66 patients treated. This was more likely in patients with gastrointestinal ulceration, trauma to a blood vessel, injury of a vascular organ, or highly abnormal coagulation (low platelets, raised PT, and APTT), for example in liver disease.

The role of bacterial gut translocation in multiple organ failure

All the inotropes described above have been studied with regard to their effect on the splanchnic circulation. Gastric mucosal pH can be measured using nasogastric probes and is thought to be a marker of perfusion in this particular vascular bed. A fall in gastric mucosal pH indicates vasoconstriction and reduced perfusion. Compromised perfusion allows breakdown of the mucosal barrier, and gut bacteria pass into the portal circulation. Bacteria and endotoxin come into direct contact with Kupffer cells in the liver, stimulating cytokine production and release. These mediators spill over into the systemic circulation and lead to organ dysfunction. This theory has been demonstrated in animal studies, but the role of bacterial gut translocation in the development of multiple organ failure in humans is still an area of research. There is a great interest in nutrition, immunonutrition, and the effects of various vasoactive drugs on the splanchnic circulation for this reason.

Microbiological considerations

Once resuscitation is underway, an attempt should be made to isolate the cause of severe sepsis. In many cases, this involves the hunt for an infective organism using serial blood cultures and imaging. This is an important aspect of management as intervention, such as the drainage of an abscess, can improve the course of illness more effectively than antibiotics alone. Serial C-reactive protein or procalcitonin measurements are useful markers in severe sepsis. Procalcitonin is thought to be more specific in differentiating bacterial from non-bacterial inflammation and may be of value in the initiation of empirical antibiotic therapy. Bacterial infections are the commonest aetiological agents of both community-acquired and hospital-related sepsis (Figure 7.4), but a causative organism is confirmed in only 60% cases. Disease progression is similar regardless of organism. However, there has been a rise in multiply resistant bacteria such as *Acinobacter* species, *Enterococci* and methicillin-resistant *Staphylococcus aureus* (MRSA).

Retrospective studies have shown that early administration of appropriate antibiotics reduces the mortality of patients with Gram negative bacteraemia and it is likely that appropriate antibiotic therapy also reduces the morbidity and mortality in Gram positive sepsis. The choice of antibiotic should take into account history, examination, and microbiological investigations. "Blind" antibiotic therapy is often started in severely ill patients based on history and examination alone (Table 7.2).

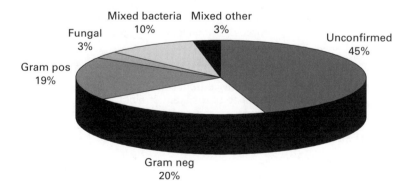

Figure 7.4 Pathogens in sepsis

Table 7.2 UK "blind" antibiotic therapy in severe sepsis (policies vary between institutions)

Symptoms and signs	Likely organisms	Intravenous therapy
Severe community-acquired pneumonia	*Pneumococcus*, *Mycoplasma*, *Legionella*	Cefuroxime + erythromycin (high dose erythromycin +/− rifampicin for *Legionella*)
Hospital-acquired pneumonia	*Staphylococcus aureus*, mixed anaerobes, Gram negative rods	Cefotaxime (take into account antibiotic/ICU history and sputum cultures)
Intra-abdominal sepsis (e.g. postoperative or peritonitis)	Gram negative bacteria, anaerobes	Cefuroxime and metronidazole +/− gentamicin
Pyelonephritis	*Escherichia, coli, Enterobacter*	Cefotaxime or ciprofloxacin
Meningitis	*Pneumococcus, Meningococcus*	Cefotaxime
Meningitis in patients aged over 50	*Pneumococcus, Meningococcus, Listeria*, Gram negative rods	Cefotaxime + ampicillin
Neutropenic patients (e.g. from chemotherapy)	*Staphylococcus aureus, Pseudomonas, Klebsiella, Escherichia coli*	Piperacillin-tazobactam + gentamicin
Line infections	*Staphylococcus aureus*, Gram negative bacteria	Replace line if possible. Flucloxacillin + gentamicin or vancomycin
Bone – osteomyelitis or septic arthritis	*Staphylococcus aureus*	Flucloxacillin +/− fucidic acid
Acute endocarditis	*Staphylococcus aureus*, Gram negative bacteria, *Streptococcus viridans*	Benzylpenicillin + gentamicin
Returning traveller	Seek advice from consultant microbiologist because of resistant strains	

Note: If there is serious penicillin or cephalosporin allergy, consult urgently with microbiologist.

Box 7.3 Microbiological investigations in severe sepsis

Initial tests
- Blood count, urea and electrolytes, liver tests, clotting screen, glucose, and CRP
- Repeated blood cultures, urine culture, chest x ray
- Serology and PCR tests (take advice)

Chest signs
- Sputum culture or bronchoscopy + lavage

CNS signs
- Brain CT +/− lumbar puncture

Abdominal signs, postabdominal surgery or no obvious cause of sepsis
- Abdominal ultrasound + CT

Heart murmur
- Echocardiogram

The most common radiological investigations include chest x ray film and abdominal CT scanning (Box 7.3). Laparotomy does not improve outcome in a critically ill patient in whom radiological examination has failed to show a surgically correctable problem.

Self-assessment – case histories

1. A 52-year-old man underwent an elective colonoscopy for investigation of constipation. Two hours later he developed severe abdominal pain and vomiting. The duty doctor diagnosed colonic perforation, which was confirmed by x ray film. The surgical team was informed and part of his large bowel was resected at laparotomy. Later, the patient's observations are as follows: temperature 38°C, pulse 110 per minute, RR 30 per minute, BP 90/50 mmHg and poor urine output. He is mildly confused. Investigations show: Hb 10·5 g dl^{-1}, WBC 20 × 10^9 litre^{-1}, platelets 70 × 10^9 litre^{-1}, Na 135 mmol litre^{-1}, K 4·7 mmol litre^{-1}, urea 15 mmol litre^{-1} (BUN 41·6 mg dl^{-1}), and creatinine 150 µmol litre^{-1} (1·8 mg dl^{-1}). Arterial blood gases on 5 litres per minute via a simple face mask showed: pH 7·26, PO_2 8·2 kPa (63 mmHg), PCO_2 5·3 kPa (40·7 mmHg), bicarbonate 17·5 mmol/l, BE − 8. A CVP line has been inserted after 1500 ml colloid. The initial reading is 12 mmHg. What is your further management?
2. A 50-year-old lady was seen in the Emergency Department and treated for a urinary tract infection on the basis of symptoms and

a positive urine dipstick. The next day she returned having collapsed. On arrival her observations were as follows: alert, pulse 120 per minute, temperature 38°C, BP 80/50 mmHg, RR 20 per minute, SaO_2 95% on air, urine output normal. What is your management and what other immediate tests do you perform?

3. A 19-year-old intravenous drug user was admitted with a severe hand infection secondary to injecting with dirty needles. His hand and arm were becoming increasingly swollen. He is alert but his other observations are: BP 70/40 mmHg, pyrexial, RR 20 per minute, SaO_2 95% on air, pulse 130 per minute. He has no peripheral venous access possible. Describe your management.

4. A 45-year-old lady with severe rheumatoid arthritis is admitted with a painful right hip. She is on monthly infusions of immunosuppressant therapy for her rheumatoid disease as well as daily steroids. Her admission blood tests show a raised C-reactive protein and neutrophil count. Her vital signs on admission are: BP 130/60 mmHg, temperature 36·7°C, RR 16 per minute, SaO_2 98% on air, and pulse 80 per minute. She is alert. However, 24 hours later she develops hypotension (BP 75/40 mmHg) and a tachycardia (110 per minute). A blood culture report is phoned through as "*Staphylococcus aureus* in both bottles". She is alert, apyrexial, with a respiratory rate of 24 per minute and SaO_2 of 87% on air. What is your management?

5. A 50-year-old man is admitted with pneumonia. He is seen by a junior doctor and prescribed intravenous antibiotics and fluids. When you review him, his vital signs are as follows: BP 90/50 mmHg, pulse 100 per minute, RR 30 per minute, SaO_2 85% on 5 litres per minute via a simple face mask, temperature 39°C, and he is alert. What do you do next?

6. A 40-year-old man is admitted with abdominal pain, which is diagnosed as acute pancreatitis (amylase of 2000 units litre^{-1}). He is given a high concentration of oxygen, intravenous fluids, and analgesia. Six hours later he develops a poor urine output. His vital signs are: BP 95/60 mmHg, pulse 120 per minute, RR 25 per minute, SaO_2 90% on 10 litres per minute via a reservoir bag mask, temperature 38°C, and he is alert. Blood lactate is 2·8 mmol litre^{-1} (normal 0·7–1·2 mmol litre^{-1}). What is your management?

7. A 60-year-old lady develops a poor urine output following an emergency endoscopic retrograde cholesytopancreatogram (ERCP) for common bile duct stones and ascending cholangitis. Her vital signs are: BP 100/75 mmHg, pulse 80 per minute, RR 20 per minute, SaO_2 97% on air, temperature 37·5°C, and she is alert. What is your management?

8. A 30-year-old man is admitted with a severe gastrointestinal bleed and receives 14 units of packed red blood cells plus other colloids during 4 hours of stabilisation followed by upper gastrointestinal endoscopy. He is then transferred to theatre for surgical repair of a large bleeding duodenal ulcer. Twenty four hours after surgery

he is still ventilated and has increasing oxygen requirements. A chest x ray film shows bilateral patchy infiltrates. His vital signs are: BP 110/70 mmHg, pulse 110 per minute, RR 14 per minute (ventilated), SaO_2 95% on 60% oxygen, temperature 37°C. What is the diagnosis and what is your management?

9. A 29-year-old lady arrives in the resuscitation room drowsy with the following vital signs: BP 80/50 mmHg, pulse 130 per minute, RR 28 per minute, SaO_2 95% on 10 litres per minute via a reservoir bag mask, temperature 38·5°C. Her arterial blood gases show: pH 7·3, PaO_2 35·5 kPa (273 mmHg), $PaCO_2$ 3·5 (26·9 mmHg), bicarbonate 12·7 mmol/l, BE − 10. She has a petechial rash on her trunk. She responds to voice. Her bedside glucose measurement is 6·2 mmol litre^{-1} (103 mg dl^{-1}) and there is no neck stiffness. What is your management?

Self-assessment − discussion

1. Bacterial peritonitis has caused severe sepsis. Mortality associated with perforation varies according to site − < 5% for small bowel and appendix, 10% for the gastroduodenal tract, 20–30% for the colon, and 50% for postoperative anastomotic leaks. This man has signs of organ dysfunction, hypoperfusion (low BP, urine output, and metabolic acidosis), and possibly DIC. The $PaCO_2$ is normal, though a compensatory respiratory alkalosis is expected. This is because he is unable to maintain a high minute volume indefinitely and is tiring. The immediate management includes ensuring a patent airway and administering a high concentration of oxygen. Assessment of breathing includes looking for signs of ARDS (note his PaO_2 of 8·2 − a chest x ray film is indicated). For circulation, intravenous access followed by repeated fluid challenges is required. Intravenous analgesia should not be forgotten. Since the cause of the sepsis is known, appropriate antibiotics can be given. The initial CVP reading is 12 mmHg, but fluid should still be given because it is the response to a fluid challenge, not a single reading, that allows interpretation of the CVP and volume status. If the patient is adequately filled but still hypotensive and oliguric, a vasopressor should be administered to increase renal perfusion pressure. Early referral to the ICU team is imperative.

2. Immediate management in this case includes assessment of the airway and giving a high concentration of oxygen (for example, 15 litres per minute via a reservoir bag mask), examining the chest, and an assessment of the circulation (pulse, blood pressure, skin temperature, etc.). She is alert. Immediate tests in acutely ill patients always consist of arterial blood gases and a bedside glucose measurement. As intravenous access is required, blood cultures, haematology, and biochemistry can be taken at the same time. The likeliest source of sepsis in this case is the urine and this should be cultured. Successive fluid challenges are required to restore organ perfusion and the attending doctor

should stay with the patient until satisfied that this is the case but, if this fails, the patient should be referred to the ICU for treatment with vasoactive drugs.

3. Again this patient needs assessment and treatment of A, B, C – high concentration oxygen and several fluid challenges in this case. A CVP line is indicated immediately because of his lack of peripheral venous access. The swelling could be cellulitis, but search also for soft tissue crepitus. The presence of a rapidly progressing site of infection with severe systemic symptoms and signs is suggestive of necrotising fasciitis, which requires urgent surgical debridement as well as intravenous antibiotics. Check the creatinine kinase levels as the patient may also be developing compartment syndrome with rhabdomyolysis.

4. Check A, B, and C. The airway is secure. Examination of breathing reveals a respiratory rate of 24 per minute and low oxygen saturations (87% on air). Oxygen therapy is required, for example 15 litres per minute via a reservoir bag mask. In the circulation, fluid challenges are required in order to treat hypoperfusion. However, capillary leak and other changes in the lung mean that pulmonary oedema can develop with normal left ventricular function. If fluid loading does not improve blood pressure and perfusion, invasive monitoring and vasopressors are required. In this case the source of sepsis is known (staphylococcal septic arthritis) and high dose intravenous antibiotics should be given. Advice should be taken on surgical drainage of the affected hip. If she is on a significant dose of long-term steroids, these will need to be increased. The low oxygen saturations and high respiratory rate could indicate the development of ARDS. Taken together, these signs indicate severe sepsis and consideration should be given to the aggressive prevention of full blown multiple organ dysfunction syndrome. This patient requires early admission to ICU. Mortality increases with increasing organ failure (Table 7.3).

5. Assess the airway by asking the patient a question. If he is alert and talking, the airway is secure. Administer a higher concentration of oxygen (for example, 15 litres per minute via a

Table 7.3 Mortality and number of failing organ systems

Number of failing organs	ICU patients (%)	Mortality (%)
0	35	3
1	25	10·5
2	17	25·5
3	12	51·5
4	6·5	61
5	3·0	67
6	1·5	91

reservoir bag mask). Next, assess breathing. His respiratory rate is raised and examination of the chest will be consistent with pneumonia. Then assess circulation. Is there hypovolaemia or hypoperfusion? Fever and increased respiratory rate caused by pneumonia cause dehydration. Arterial blood gas analysis may indicate hypoperfusion. His hypotension may respond simply to a fluid challenge. If severe sepsis is present, the hypotension may not respond to fluid challenges alone. In that case, invasive monitoring is required to be sure the patient is adequately filled, followed by the use of vasoactive drugs. The patient should be referred to the ICU.

6. The management in this case is the same – A, B, C. In this patient, attention to detail may prevent the multiple systemic complications of severe acute pancreatitis, especially respiratory failure, renal failure, and infection. The classic presentation in severe cases is SIRS (systemic inflammatory response syndrome) and MODS (multiple organ dysfunction syndrome). Mortality is as high as 20–30%. This patient requires oxygen and fluid challenges immediately. Make your goals known to the nursing staff. Aim for:

- systolic BP > 100 mmHg
- CVP > 10 mmHg
- urine output > 0·5 ml kg^{-1} per hour
- reduction in lactate or base deficit.

Look for developing ARDS and the need for early ventilation. This patient requires ICU care. If the hypoperfusion does not respond to fluid challenges, invasive monitoring and vasoactive drugs are required in order to:

- restore an effective circulating volume
- restore adequate perfusion
- maintain an adequate cardiac output and oxygen delivery.

7. Again, this lady requires assessment of airway, high concentration oxygen therapy, assessment of breathing and circulation followed by fluid challenges. Note that a blood pressure of 100/75 mmHg is causing hypoperfusion here – in some patients this is a normal blood pressure. Antibiotics are required. She needs referral to the ICU if fluid challenges fail to correct the hypoperfusion. How many fluid challenges would one give in this situation? At first, clinical endpoints of blood pressure, pulse, peripheral skin temperature, and respiratory rate may be used to assess volume status. However, after several fluid challenges, there is potential for fluid overload without improvement in perfusion, especially in the context of capillary leak. Invasive monitoring is then helpful in assessing volume status and in the administration of vasoactive drugs.

8. This patient has received a massive blood transfusion, which can cause ARDS. Arterial blood gases would show a large A–a

gradient from intrapulmonary shunting. The ventilator may calculate lung compliance which would be low and typical of developing acute lung injury. The management in this case is to continue invasive ventilation on the ICU. The various ventilation strategies employed are discussed in the chapter.

9. This patient has severe sepsis according to the definition at the beginning of the chapter. The arterial blood gases show a metabolic acidosis indicating hypoperfusion. Ensure a patent and protected airway, give a high concentration of oxygen (for example, 15 litres per minute via a reservoir bag mask), assess and treat any breathing problems, assess and treat any circulation problems, and assess conscious level. A full examination and appropriate investigations (including blood and other cultures) should follow. In this case, fluid challenges are required. The petechial rash is a clue to the possible cause of sepsis and intravenous antibiotics should be given to cover meningococcal and staphylococcal infections.

Further reading

Bernard GR, Artigas A, Brigham KL *et al*. The American-European Consensus Conference on ARDS. *Am J Respir Crit Care Med* 1994;**149**:818–24.

Busund R, Koukline V, Utrobin U, Nedashkovsky E. Plasmapheresis in severe sepsis and septic shock: a prospective randomised controlled trial. *Intens Care Med* 2002;**28**:1434–9.

Reinhart K, Sakka SG, Meier-Hellmann A. Haemodynamic management of a patient with septic shock. *Eur J Anaesthesiol* 2000;**17**:6–17.

Rivers E, Nguyen B, Havstad S *et al*. Early goal-directed therapy in the treatment of severe sepsis and septic shock. *New Engl J Med* 2001;**345**: 1368–77.

8: Acute renal failure

By the end of this chapter you will be able to:

- appreciate that prevention is better than cure
- understand the important physiological factors in renal perfusion
- know the evidence – or lack of it – behind various treatments for acute renal failure
- understand the principles of renal replacement therapy
- apply this to your clinical practice

Preventing renal failure

Acute renal failure is defined as acute oliguria (< 400 ml per day) or a rapid (hours to weeks) decline in glomerular filtration rate manifested by a rise in urea and creatinine. The rise in creatinine is often slow. In fact, if all renal function is lost, the serum creatinine rises by only 80–160 µmol litre⁻¹ (1–2 mg dl⁻¹) per day. Oliguria is defined as the production of 100–400 ml urine per day. Anuria is defined as the production of < 100 ml per day, whilst absolute anuria is no urine output. Absolute anuria reflects urinary tract obstruction until proven otherwise. It is generally believed that a urine output of < 0·5 ml kg⁻¹ per hour for greater than two hours is an important marker of renal hypoperfusion and should trigger remedial action. However, 50–60% of acute renal failure is non-oliguric.

Hypotension, dehydration, and sepsis are the commonest causes of acute tubular necrosis. Prerenal causes of acute renal failure are the most common in both hospital and the community (Box 8.1). Overall mortality from unselected cases of acute renal failure has remained at around 50% (70% on ICU). Mortality increases with serum creatinine: 5–20% < 165 µmol litre⁻¹ (2 mg dl⁻¹) and 64% over 250 µmol litre⁻¹ (3 mg dl⁻¹). Mortality has not changed significantly in over 20 years, making prevention of acute renal failure a high priority. Even with the advent of renal replacement therapy, the change in case mix, increasing age of patients, and severity of underlying conditions may help to explain the static mortality rate. Overall it is estimated that 5% hospital admissions and 30%

Box 8.1 Causes of acute renal failure

- Acute tubular necrosis – 45%
- Prerenal causes – 21%
- New onset chronic renal failure – 13%
- Obstruction – 10%
- Glomerulonephritis 3%
- Acute tubulo-interstitial nephritis 2%
- Vasculitis 1·5%
- Other 3·5%

---

intensive care admissions have acute renal failure and 2–5% hospitalised patients develop it; 30% patients with acute renal failure will need renal replacement therapy.

The kidney is especially vulnerable to injury resulting from hypoperfusion and/or critical illness. A study by Hou *et al.* in 1993 looked at all patients admitted to medicine and surgery in their hospital over a 6-month period (excluding those with renal failure). Patients were screened during their stay for worsening of renal function: 5% of these patients developed renal insufficiency – 42% because of hypoperfusion (of these hypotension 41%, major cardiac dysfunction 30%, and sepsis 19%). Major surgery accounted for 18%, contrast media 12%, aminoglycoside administration 7%, and miscellaneous causes 21% (for example, obstruction). The severity of renal insufficiency as judged by serum creatinine was the most important indicator of a poor prognosis. The overall mortality rate was 25% – but this rose to 64% in those patients with an increase in creatinine of 265 μmol litre^{-1} (3·18 mg dl^{-1}) or more.

Mortality is especially high in acute renal failure in those patients who have had a myocardial infarction or stroke, have oliguria, sepsis, are male, elderly, or are mechanically ventilated. Patients at risk of acute renal failure can be identified, and hypoperfusion and obstruction can be treated early, so it is likely that a proportion of mortality from acute renal failure is preventable. The reality is that much hypoperfusion is left untreated for several hours and incorrect treatment leads to further deterioration, causing irreversible renal failure.

It is imperative that early effective action is taken to prevent permanent renal failure as soon as renal function becomes compromised.

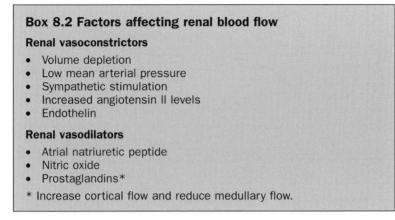

Box 8.2 Factors affecting renal blood flow

Renal vasoconstrictors

- Volume depletion
- Low mean arterial pressure
- Sympathetic stimulation
- Increased angiotensin II levels
- Endothelin

Renal vasodilators

- Atrial natriuretic peptide
- Nitric oxide
- Prostaglandins*

* Increase cortical flow and reduce medullary flow.

Renal blood flow

Renal blood flow is normally 1200 ml per minute, just over 20% cardiac output. It is affected by various factors (Box 8.2).

There is autoregulation of renal blood flow between a MAP of 70–170 in normal subjects (autoregulation in hypertensive patients is shifted to the right, Figure 8.1). Resistance of the renal vascular bed plays a large part in autoregulation – the smooth muscle walls of the afferent and efferent arterioles in the cortex constrict and dilate according to changes in pressure. Renal artery perfusion depends on a critical perfusion pressure.

$$\text{Renal blood flow} = \frac{\text{input pressure} - \text{output pressure}}{\text{resistance of renal vascular bed}}$$

that is, renal blood flow is maintained, within the limits of autoregulation, by changing the pressure gradient and resistance of the vascular bed.

The kidney is one of the most highly perfused organs in the body. In other organs, as blood flow falls, oxygen extraction increases but, in the kidney, oxygen consumption falls in parallel with blood flow. Initially the afferent (input) vessels dilate and the efferent (output) vessels constrict, to try and maintain an effective perfusion pressure to produce a glomerular filtrate. Total renal oxygen consumption is low except in the outer medulla where active sodium reabsorption occurs. Frusemide blocks the active sodium–potassium–chloride cotransport system in the thick ascending limb of the

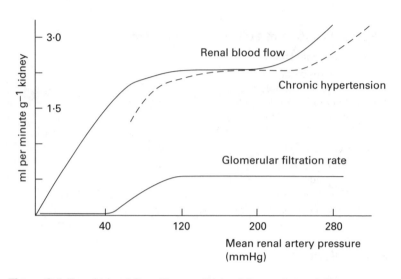

Figure 8.1 Renal blood flow. The renal blood flow autoregulation curve is shifted to the right in chronic hypertension

loop of Henle (Figure 8.2). This area is normally relatively hypoxic because of high tubular reabsorptive activity. In rats, frusemide abolishes the physiological outer medullary hypoxia despite a fall in blood flow but this has failed to translate into a benefit in clinical practice.

Estimating renal function

Neither urine output nor creatinine are good estimates of renal function. Creatinine clearance is more helpful and can be estimated by the equation:

$$\text{Clearance} = \frac{(140 - \text{age}) \times \text{weight in kg}}{\text{creatinine in } \mu\text{mol litre}^{-1}} \; (\times 1.2 \text{ for men})$$

Normal is around 100 ml per minute but this formula was derived for use in the steady state and, if the creatinine is rising, true clearance will be lower. In oedematous patients, the GFR can be overestimated as total body weight is greater than lean body mass. However, it is useful and can provide guidance for drug adjustments. Particularly in the elderly, with less muscle mass, "normal" creatinines can be deceptive. If an 80-year-old man of 60 kg has a creatinine of 100 μmol litre^{-1}

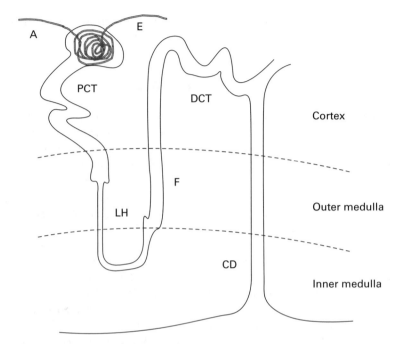

Figure 8.2 The nephron (the functional unit of the kidney). A, afferent arteriole where ACE inhibitors act (angiotensin II plays a role in autoregulation of renal blood flow by constricting the afferent blood vessels when there are low pressures); CD, collecting duct; DCT, distal convoluted tubule; E, efferent arteriole where NSAIDs act (prostaglandins play a role in regulation of renal blood flow and increase cortical flow; in a person on ACE inhibitors and NSAIDs who is admitted with vomiting and diarrhoea – or hypovolaemia of any cause – both these drugs should be temporarily stopped; the combination of hypovolaemia, lack of constriction in the afferent vessels, and lack of vasodilatation in the efferent vessels reduces GFR; in cirrhosis and congestive cardiac failure where prostaglandins are recruited to increase renal blood flow, NSAIDs are more potent); F, thick ascending limb of the loop of Henle where frusemide blocks active sodium–potassium–chloride cotransport (despite documented protective effects in experiments, frusemide has failed to prevent postoperative renal failure in high risk patients or ameliorate established acute renal failure in clinical practice); LH, thick and thin descending and ascending Loop of Henle; PCT, proximal convoluted tubule.

(1.2 mg dl^{-1}), although this is within the "normal" range, his actual creatinine clearance is 43 ml per minute.

Pathophysiology of acute renal failure

The pathophysiology behind acute renal failure (ARF) is complex and only partly understood. Many data come from animal models where acute tubular necrosis is induced by transiently clamping a renal artery. Real patients are more complex, where renal failure is often part of a developing multisystem illness. The outer medulla is relatively hypoxic and prone to injury. When there is an ischaemic or septic insult, inflammatory mediators damage the endothelium. It is not as simple as damaged tubular cells sloughing and blocking the collecting ducts; there is a complex response Involving programmed cell death (apoptosis) and damage to the actin cytoskeleton, which facilitates cell-to-cell adhesion and forms the barrier between blood and filtrate. Genetic factors also play a role. "Knockout" mice without the gene for a cell adhesion molecule ICAM–1 (which helps leukocytes bind to the endothelium) do not develop ARF after an ischaemic insult.

Ischaemic or nephrotoxic acute tubular necrosis (ATN) accounts for 80–90% perioperative renal failure. A prospective multicentre study in Madrid in 1998 showed that out of 253 cases of acute renal failure in ICU, 76% were due to ATN, 18% due to a prerenal cause, and only two cases due to obstruction. In the critically ill, glomerulonephritis as a cause of acute renal failure is uncommon.

In animal models, interruption of blood flow for less than 25 minutes results in oliguria but no anatomical changes and renal function returns to normal; 60–120 minutes of interrupted blood flow causes tubular cell damage. These are the metabolically active cells. Renal recovery can occur if further insults are avoided. Interruption of blood blow for over 120 minutes causes renal infarction and irreversible acute renal failure. High risk surgical procedures for the development of acute renal failure are cardiac surgery, vascular surgery, biliary and hepatic surgery (because bile salts bind endotoxins, which cause renal vasoconstriction, and this action ceases in cholestasis), urological surgery, and procedures associated with intra-abdominal hypertension.

> **Box 8.3 Causes of acute renal failure**
>
> **Prerenal causes**
> - Reduced cardiac output (dysfunction or hypovolaema)
> - Redistribution of blood flow (sepsis, liver failure)
>
> **Renal causes**
> - Acute tubular necrosis (ATN) – from any prolonged prerenal cause
> - ATN from toxins (drugs, contrast media)
> - Vasculitis, myeloma, emboli, glomerulonephritis
>
> **Post-renal causes**
> - Obstruction (stones, prostate, tumours, ureteric damage during surgery)

Regardless of the cause of acute renal failure, the reduction in renal blood flow represents a common pathological pathway leading to reduced glomerular filtration. Causes of acute renal failure are traditionally divided into three groups (Box 8.3).

During the period of reduced renal blood flow, the kidneys are particularly vulnerable to further insults. At risk patients are those with diabetes, vascular disease, known renal impairment, with a recent major upset such as myocardial infarction, major surgery or GI bleed, and on nephrotoxic medication (in particular the combination of angiotensin converting enzyme [ACE] inhibitors and non-steroidal anti-inflammatory drugs [NSAIDs]) and also drugs such as aminoglycosides, allopurinol, and digoxin. Up to 25% hospital patients receiving therapeutic aminoglycosides sustain some degree of renal impairment.

Recovery from acute renal failure does not just depend only on restoration of renal blood flow, although early restoration leads to improved outcome. In intrinsic renal failure, once renal blood flow is restored, the remaining functional nephrons increase their filtration and hypertrophy. Recovery is dependent on the number of remaining functional nephrons. If this is below a critical value, continued hyperfiltration results in progressive glomerular sclerosis, which eventually leads to nephron loss. Continued nephron loss causes more hyperfiltration until renal failure results. This has been termed the hyperfiltration theory of renal failure, and it explains why progressive renal failure is sometimes observed after apparent recovery from acute renal failure.

Table 8.1 Measurements which may point towards the cause of acute renal failure

Parameters	Prerenal	Renal
Urine osmolality (mmol litre^{-1})	> 500	< 350
Fractional excretion of Na (%)*	< 1	> 4
Urine Na (mmol litre^{-1})	< 20	> 40
Urine:plasma creatinine ratio	> 40	< 10

$$\frac{*\text{Urine Na/serum Na}}{\text{Urine creatinine/serum creatinine}} \times 100$$

There are various urine tests that can help point towards renal or prerenal causes (Table 8.1). This is based on the fact that in prerenal failure the kidney avidly reabsorbs salt and water, but in renal failure where tubular function is disrupted, the kidney loses sodium in the urine. In practice these are not much help in patients already in hospital where there is often a clear precipitating cause. Diuretics also increase the urinary excretion of sodium and this makes urinary sodium values difficult to interpret.

Treatment of acute renal failure

Early action saves kidneys. The principles of treatment are as follows:

- Treat any life-threatening hyperkalaemia first.
- Correct hypovolaemia and establish an effective circulating volume.
- Treat hypoperfusion.
- Exclude obstruction as soon as possible.
- Treat the underlying cause.

In acute renal failure, early restoration of volume may be all that is required. Sometimes, volume replacement fails to restore blood pressure (for example, in severe sepsis or acute cardiac failure) in which case vasoactive drugs are required to improve renal perfusion. Bicarbonate should not be given to treat a metabolic acidosis that is due to hypoperfusion. After

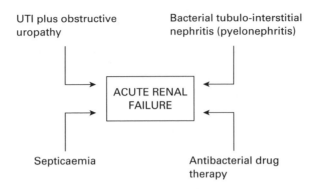

Figure 8.3 Acute renal failure caused by urinary tract infection (UTI). There is evidence to suggest a direct effect on the kidney by endotoxins. Dehydration owing to vomiting and NSAID use also contribute. Pre-existing renal impairment or diabetes increases risk. Reprinted with permission of Oxford University Press (*Advanced Renal Medicine*, by AEG Raine, 1992)

volume restoration, fluid may be restricted to measurable plus insensible losses to avoid volume overload in oliguric patients. Frusemide is often used at his point. If the patient fails to respond to restoration of volume and perfusion, renal replacement therapy (RRT) is the next step. Patients require RRT for an average of 13 days and around 36% patients with acute renal failure require this. Only 3% require RRT long term. Liaison with a renal specialist is important.

Non-obstructive urinary tract infection is an important cause of acute renal failure, sometimes overlooked, and should be aggressively treated (Figure 8.3).

Many treatments improve urine output but have no effect on outcome in established ARF:

- high dose loop diuretics (bolus or infusion)
- mannitol
- dopamine.

Frusemide is said to cause a reduction in renal oxygen demand and mannitol is thought to scavenge free radicals – theoretical benefits that are not borne out in clinical practice. However, loop diuretics can help convert oliguric renal failure to non-oliguric renal failure and thus avoid problems with volume overload.

There are many potential treatments that have been tried in the prevention of ARF and have been found to be ineffective:

- frusemide
- mannitol
- dopamine and dopexamine
- other experimental treatments (for example, theophylline and acetylcysteine).

Mini-tutorial: low dose dopamine in acute renal failure

Using low dose dopamine at 0·2–2·5 micrograms kg^{-1} per minute ("renal dose") for both the prevention and treatment of acute renal failure is common. Yet randomised trials have shown it is of no benefit either as prevention in high risk postoperative patients or as treatment in established acute renal failure. The effects of a dopamine infusion are complicated because it acts on a number of different receptors that have opposing actions. The action of dopamine is not constant throughout its dose range (see a fuller description in Chapter 6). Stimulation of α receptors causes systemic vasoconstriction and the blood pressure rises; β1 receptors increase contractility of the heart, β2 receptors reduce afterload, and dopamine (DA) receptors cause renal and splanchnic vasodilatation. Dopamine acts on all these receptors. In addition, there are two major subgroups of DA receptor: DA1 receptors are in the renal and mesenteric circulation; DA2 receptors are in the autonomic ganglia and sympathetic nerve endings and inhibit noradrenaline release. Dopamine and its synthetic sister dopexamine have been used extensively to theoretically improve renal blood flow and therefore function. Dopexamine is also used to improve splanchnic blood flow in certain postoperative situations.

Dopamine causes a diuresis and natriuresis independent of any effect on renal blood flow by inhibiting proximal tubule Na–K–ATPase (via DA1 and DA2 stimulation). So the effect we see with low dose dopamine is a diuresis – not a change in creatinine clearance. In one randomised prospective double-blind trial, 23 patients at risk for renal dysfunction were given either dopamine at 200 micrograms per minute, dobutamine at 175 micrograms per minute, or 5% dextrose. Dopamine increased urine output without a change in creatinine clearance and dobutamine caused a significant increase in creatinine clearance by increasing cardiac output without an increase in urine output. This illustrates the difficulty of using urine output as a surrogate marker for renal function.

Critically ill patients have reduced dopamine clearance and may consequently have higher plasma levels than anticipated, so it is not correct to assume that low dose dopamine is acting only on the renal circulation. In one study, there was a 27-fold variability in the range of plasma dopamine levels. In some individuals, infusion of "renal dose" dopamine results in plasma levels in the α-receptor range. This leads to side effects such as tachyarrhythmias and increased afterload. In summary, there is no evidence to justify the use of dopamine to prevent or treat acute renal failure.

Renal replacement therapy – haemodialysis and haemofiltration

Indications for RRT in acute renal failure are as follows:

- hyperkalaemia especially if ECG changes
- volume overload
- worsening severe metabolic acidosis
- uraemic complications, for example encephalopathy, pericarditis, and seizures.

Haemodialysis removes solutes from blood by their passage across a semipermeable membrane. Heparinised blood flows in one direction and dialysis fluid flows in another at a faster rate. Dialysis fluid contains physiological levels of electrolytes except potassium, which is low, and molecules cross the membrane by simple diffusion along a concentration gradient. Smaller molecules move faster than larger ones. Urea and creatinine concentrations are zero in the dialysis fluid because they are to be removed as much as possible. A 3–4-hour treatment can reduce urea by 70%. Water can be removed by applying a pressure gradient across the membrane if needed.

Haemofiltration involves blood under pressure moving down one side of a semipermeable membrane. This has a similar effect to glomerular filtration, and small and large molecules are cleared at the same rates. Instead of selective reabsorption, which occurs in the kidney, the whole filtrate is discarded and the patient is infused with a replacement physiological solution instead (Box 8.4). Less fluid may be replaced than is removed in cases of fluid overload. In original haemofiltration, the femoral artery and vein were cannulated (continuous arteriovenous haemofiltration or CAVH). Blood

> **Box 8.4 Typical composition of haemofiltration replacement fluid (mmol litre^{-1})**
>
> - Sodium – 140
> - Potassium – Variable and added just before use
> - Calcium – 1·6
> - Magnesium – 0·75
> - Chloride – 101
> - Lactate – 45
> - Glucose – 11

passed through the filter under arterial pressure alone – but circuit disconnection could lead to rapid blood loss and patients with low blood pressures often had slow moving circuits with the associated risk of blood clotting. In more common use today is continuous venovenous haemofiltration or CVVH. A large vein is cannulated using a double lumen catheter and a pump controls blood flow. The extracorporeal circuit is anticoagulated in both CAVH and CVVH. Automated systems have a replacement fluid pump that can either balance input and output or allow a programmed rate of fluid loss.

Haemofiltration removes virtually all ions from plasma including calcium and bicarbonate. Replacing these is difficult, since solutions containing enough of these two ions can precipitate. Lactate is commonly used instead of bicarbonate but, although in normal people lactate is converted to bicarbonate, this is not true of patients with lactic acidosis. In these situations bicarbonate infusions must be given separately. Haemofiltration has advantages over haemodialysis in the critical care setting because such patients cannot be fluid restricted and often have a compromised circulation. CVVH avoids the hypotension often seen in dialysis, is continuous so it can remove large volumes of water in patients receiving parenteral nutrition and other infusions, offers better clearance of urea and solutes, may better preserve cerebral perfusion pressure, and also has a role in clearing inflammatory mediators.

The differences between haemodialysis and haemofiltration are shown in Figure 8.4.

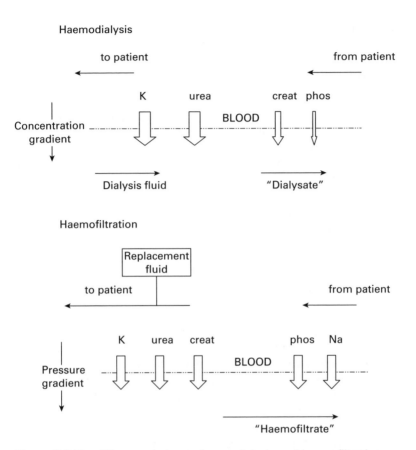

Figure 8.4 The difference between haemodialysis and haemofiltration. creat, creatinine; K, potassium; Na, sodium; phos, phosphorus

Rhabdomyloysis

Certain situations warrant the use of diuretics early in acute renal failure after restoration of intravascular volume. These are rhabdomyolysis and poisoning (for example, lithium, theophylline and salicylates). Rhabdomyolysis is an important cause of acute renal failure. It occurs when there is massive breakdown of muscle. Myoglobin is released into the circulation along with other toxins, which leads to kidney dysfunction and general metabolic upset. Unlike many other causes of acute renal failure, prognosis is good in rhabdomyolysis and the kidneys usually recover. This makes it an important condition not to miss. Causes include:

- crush injury/reperfusion after compartment syndrome
- prolonged immobility following a fall or overdose especially with hypothermia
- drug overdose, for example Ecstasy and carbon monoxide poisoning
- extreme exertion
- myositis (caused by illnesses like influenza, severe hypokalaemia or drugs like statins)
- malignant hyperthermia (triggered by some anaesthetic agents)
- neuroleptic malignant syndrome
- heat-stroke.

Myoglobin and urate from muscle breakdown are said to obstruct the tubules. Yet tubular obstruction is probably not what causes acute renal failure in rhabdomyolysis, because studies show that intratubular pressures are normal. More likely is free radical mediated injury. Renal vasoconstriction also occurs, partly because of the underlying cause and partly because myoglobin itself causes vasoconstriction.

Fluid resuscitation remains the most important aspect of management in rhabdomyolysis. Early and aggressive intravenous fluid has dramatic benefits on outcome when compared with historical controls. Guidelines go as far as 12 litres of fluid a day to "flush" the kidneys and achieve a urine output of 200–300 ml h^{-1}. Alkalinisation of the urine significantly improves renal function, probably by inhibiting free radical mediated damage. The urine is dipsticked every hour and sodium bicarbonate is given intravenously to raise the urine pH to 7·0. Mannitol is the first-line diuretic in rhabdomyolysis, but it has not been shown to be better than volume diuresis alone. Frusemide acidifies the urine but is sometimes administered after a trial of mannitol. Plasmapheresis is not an established therapy in rhabdomyolysis, although myoglobin can be removed from the circulation this way.

Self-assessment – case histories

1. A 30-year-old man was admitted after being found lying on the floor of his apartment. He had taken intravenous heroin the night before. His admission blood results showed a normal full blood count, sodium 130 mmol litre^{-1}, potassium 6 mmol litre^{-1}, urea 64 mmol litre^{-1} (blood urea nitrogen [BUN] 177 mg dl^{-1}) and creatinine 500 µmol litre^{-1} (6 mg dl^{-1}). His vital signs were: drowsiness, blood pressure 90/60 mmHg, pulse 100 per minute, respiratory rate 8 per minute and oxygen saturations 95% on air. What is your management?

2. A 60-year-old man was admitted with a general deterioration in health. He is treated for heart failure and is taking the following medication: ramipril 10 mg, frusemide 80 mg, and allopurinol 300 mg at night. He had been treated for a chest infection and pleurisy the week before admission with antibiotics (amoxycillin) and a NSAID. On examination he was drowsy and appeared dehydrated. His blood pressure was 70/40 mmHg, pulse 90 per minute, and regular, respiratory rate 25 per minute. His blood results showed: sodium 133 mmol litre^{-1}, potassium 5·0 mmol litre^{-1}, urea 50 mmol litre^{-1} (BUN 138 mg dl^{-1}), creatinine 600 µmol litre^{-1} (7·2 mg dl^{-1}). His last blood tests in hospital were a year ago, which showed a urea of 7 mmol litre^{-1} (BUN 19·4 mg dl^{-1}), and creatinine 100 µmol litre^{-1} (1·2 mg dl^{-1}). Discuss your management.

3. A 34-year-old lady was admitted with breathlessness, which had started one week ago. The chest x ray film showed bilateral patchy shadowing and she reported coughing up blood the day before admission. Her blood results showed a normal full blood count, sodium 135 mmol litre^{-1}, potassium 4·2 mmol litre^{-1}, urea 40 mmol litre^{-1} (BUN 111 mg dl^{-1}), and creatinine 450 µmol litre^{-1} (5·4 mg dl^{-1}). Her vital signs were: alert, blood pressure 180/85 mmHg, pulse 80 per minute, respiratory rate 20 per minute, and oxygen saturations 95% on air. What is your management?

4. You are asked to see a 55-year-old man on the ward. He is being treated for ascending cholangitis and had a failed endoscopic retrograde cholangiopancreatogram (ERCP) that day for treatment of a stone in the common bile duct. His vital signs are: alert, blood pressure 80/60 mmHg, pulse 80 per minute, respiratory rate 30 per minute, temperature 38°C, and oxygen saturations 96% on air. He has warm hands and feet. His medication chart shows a β blocker, calcium channel blocker, and a nitrate for angina. He has been given gentamicin intravenously for his infection. He also has a left nephrectomy scar from 15 years ago. The nurse alerts you to his urine output, which has been 10 ml h^{-1} for the last 2 hours. What is your management?

5. A 60-year-old lady is admitted with diarrhoea and vomiting, which she has had for 4 days. She has been taking a NSAID for aches and pains during the course of this illness. Her usual medication

includes bendrofluazide for hypertension. On admission her vital signs are: alert, blood pressure 90/60 mmHg, pulse 100 per minute, respiratory rate 28 per minute, and oxygen saturations 98% on air. She reports that she is passing less urine. Her blood results show: sodium 145 mmol litre^{-1}, potassium 4·0 mmol litre^{-1}, urea 25 mmol litre^{-1} (BUN 69 mg dl^{-1}) and creatinine 300 µmol litre^{-1} (3·6 mg dl^{-1}). From her records, her urea and creatinine were normal one month ago. Discuss your management.

6. An 80-year-old lady is admitted after a fractured neck of femur. She receives non-steroidal anti-inflammatory analgesia in the perioperative period. On admission her urea is 6 mmol litre^{-1} (BUN 16·6 mg dl^{-1}), and creatinine 55 µmol litre^{-1} (0·66 mg dl^{-1}). Two days postoperatively her blood results are as follows: sodium 130 mmol litre^{-1}, potassium 3·8 mmol litre^{-1}, urea 20 mmol litre^{-1} (BUN 55·5 mg dl^{-1}), and creatinine 250 µmol litre^{-1} (3 mg dl^{-1}). Her vital signs are: alert, blood pressure 180/80 mmHg, pulse 75 per minute, respiratory rate 14 per minute, and oxygen saturations 95% on air. Can you explain the cause of her acute renal failure and discuss your management?

7. A 50-year-old man with mild diabetic nephropathy is admitted to the coronary care with a myocardial infarction. He suffers a ventricular fibrillation arrest and has no pulse for 5 minutes. He has a 2-hour episode of hypotension following this, which is treated with fluid and vasoactive drugs. Although his cardiac condition recovers, his renal function worsens. On admission his urea was 12 mmol litre^{-1} (33·3 mg dl^{-1}), and creatinine 150 µmol litre^{-1} (1·8 mg dl^{-1}). Now his urea is 22 mmol litre^{-1} (61 mg dl^{-1}) and creatinine 300 µmol litre^{-1} (3·6 mg dl^{-1}). What are the reasons for his deteriorating renal function and what is your management?

8. A 55-year-old lady undergoes an elective abdominal aortic aneurysm repair. The aneurysm was located above the renal arteries and the aorta was cross-clamped for 10 minutes. She returns to the ICU from theatre still intubated. Her vital signs are: pulse 100 per minute, blood pressure 120/60 mmHg, CVP 8 mmHg, temperature 34°C. Her arterial blood gases on 40% oxygen show: pH 7·2, $PaCO_2$ 4·0 (30·7 mmHg), bicarbonate 11·5 mmol/l, BE − 12 PaO_2 25·0 kPa (192 mmHg). Her urine output has been 20 ml h^{-1} for the last 2 hours. Discuss your management.

Self-assessment – discussion

1. Any airway and breathing problems should be assessed and treated first. It may be that this patient requires naloxone to improve his conscious level and respiratory rate. Emergency treatment of hyperkalaemia is always indicated above 6·5 mmol litre^{-1} or if there are changes on the 12-lead ECG. The blood pressure of 90/60 and tachycardia could indicate volume depletion so fluid should be given to restore intravascular volume. Treatment with vasoactive drugs may be needed if

perfusion is inadequate despite volume replacement. The patient should be catheterised to allow hourly measurements of urine. An urgent renal tract ultrasound should be arranged. Finally, one should look for a treatable underlying cause. In this case, creatinine kinase should be measured as the combination of a drug overdose and prolonged immobilisation is a classical cause of rhabdomyolysis.

2. The combination of dehydration from a chest infection and medication (ACE inhibitor and NSAIDs) has triggered acute renal failure. Hypotension is causing hypoperfusion of the kidneys and making the renal impairment worse. Oxygen should be given, followed by fluid challenges to expand intravascular volume. In a patient normally treated for heart failure, invasive monitoring may be considered earlier than in people with normal cardiac function. Once intravascular volume is adequately replaced, vasopressors may be necessary to treat ongoing hypotension. He should be catheterised and a renal tract ultrasound scan arranged. Nephrotoxic medication should be stopped. If renal function fails to improve with these measures, renal replacement therapy should be considered. As with all cases of acute renal failure, urine should be sent for microscopy and culture. More specialised tests may be recommended by a renal specialist to look for other possible causes.

3. Treatment starts with an assessment of airway and breathing followed by circulation. Intravenous fluid should be given to correct any volume depletion. There is unlikely to be hypoperfusion in this case as the blood pressure is 180/85 mmHg, but other signs of this should be assessed. She should be catheterised to allow accurate measurement of urine output and an urgent renal tract ultrasound arranged. The underlying cause should be investigated. Dipstick testing, microscopy, and culture of the urine should be requested. This gives clues in conditions such as glomerulonephritis (microscopic haematuria and proteinuria) and acute tubulo-interstitial nephritis (eosinophiluria), and diagnoses urinary tract infection, which is an important cause of acute renal failure, especially in the elderly. Although the combination of breathlessness with bilateral patchy shadowing and acute renal failure may be due to chest infection and dehydration/medication as in case 2, one should consider a pulmonary-renal syndrome, for example Goodpasture's (anti-GBM disease). A renal specialist should be contacted.

4. After assessing A and B, blood cultures may be taken at the same time as gaining intravenous access. Assuming there is no life-threatening hyperkalaemia, fluid challenges should be given to treat volume depletion. Invasive monitoring may be needed if there is any uncertainty as to when the patient is adequately filled in the presence of persisting hypotension/hypoperfusion. Any anti-hypertensive medication should be temporarily stopped (apart from β blockers, which can be reduced). This patient is at

high risk of acute renal failure because of oliguria, cholestasis (which causes renal vasoconstriction), gentamicin therapy, and a previous nephrectomy – early action is essential to prevent irreversible damage to his remaining kidney. Persisting hypoperfusion despite adequate volume replacement requires vasoactive drug therapy in a high dependency area. He should be catheterised and an urgent renal ultrasound arranged. The cause of acute renal failure here is most likely to be acute tubular necrosis from hypoperfusion and sepsis.

5. The history and examination in this case point to volume depletion, which should be corrected with fluid challenges. If hypotension/hypoperfusion persists despite this, invasive monitoring and vasoactive drug therapy may be required. Note she is normally hypertensive – her normal blood pressure should be ascertained to guide therapy. She should be catheterised to allow accurate measurements of urine output. The underlying cause in this case is likely to be dehydration exacerbated by NSAID use. Frusemide is often used to improve urine output after adequate filling and perfusion has been achieved. Frusemide does not affect outcome nor alter GFR but is useful when there is persisting oliguria and the patient still requires intravenous medications. Renal replacement therapy would be the next step if there is no improvement.

6. Surgery can be associated with episodes of hypoperfusion (because of volume depletion and hypotension due to anaesthesia). Perioperative NSAID use in addition, especially in the elderly, has caused acute renal failure in this case. There is no life-threatening hyperkalaemia. Volume depletion should be treated with intravenous fluid, a urinary catheter should be inserted and a renal tract ultrasound arranged. Urinary tract infection should be excluded and nephrotoxic drugs stopped.

7. This man is at risk of developing acute renal failure because he has pre-existing diabetic renal disease and has had a major cardiovascular upset. A period of hypoperfusion has caused acute renal failure. Management is the same as in the other cases: treat any life-threatening hyperkalaemia, then hypovolaemia, then any hypoperfusion, catheterise, exclude higher obstruction with an ultrasound scan, and treat the underlying cause. If renal function continues to deteriorate, renal replacement therapy should be considered.

8. The cause of acute renal failure in this case is the transient interruption of blood flow to the renal arteries. The patient is hypoperfused as indicated by the history, low temperature, and metabolic acidosis. She should be "warmed up and filled up". Dopexamine is often used in post-aneurysm repair patients because a few small studies have suggested a beneficial effect on creatinine clearance following major surgery – probably owing to increased cardiac output and systemic vasodilatation. However, the vast majority of clinical studies of dopamine and dopexamine following major surgery have not demonstrated a benefit.

Further reading

Ball, CM and Phillips RS. Acute renal failure. In: *Acute Medicine (Evidence-based on-call series)*. London: Churchill Livingstone 2001.

Burton CJ, Tomson CRV. Can the use of low-dose dopamine for treatment of acute renal failure be justified? *Postgrad Med J* 1999;**75**:269–74.

Galley HF, ed. *Renal failure (Critical care focus series)*. London: Intensive Care Society/BMJ Books, 1999.

Hou SH, Bushinsky DA, Wish JB, Cohen JJ, Harrington JT. Hospital-acquired renal insufficiency: a prospective study. *Am J Med* 1993;**74**:243–8.

Kellum JA, Leblane M, eds. Acute renal failure. In: *Clinical Evidence*. London: BMJ Books, 2001.

Ward MM. Factors predictive of acute renal failure in rhabdomyolysis. *Arch Intern Med* 1988;**148**:1553–7.

9: Brain failure

By the end of this chapter you will be able to:

- manage the unconscious patient with confidence
- understand primary and secondary brain injury
- understand the principles of brain protection
- understand the neurological prognosis following cardiac arrest
- apply this to your clinical practice.

The unconscious patient

A reduced conscious level is common in acute illness and can be associated with potentially life-threatening complications requiring urgent intervention. Coma (or unconsciousness) is when the Glasgow Coma Scale is 8 or less (Box 9.1).

Box 9.1 Glasgow Coma Scale

Score

Eye opening

- spontaneous – 4
- to speech – 3
- to pain – 2
- nil – 1

Best motor response

- obeys commands – 6
- localises pain – 5
- withdraws to pain – 4
- abnormal flexion to pain – 3
- extensor response to pain – 2
- nil – 1

Best verbal response

- orientated – 5
- confused conversation – 4
- inappropriate words – 3
- incomprehensible sounds – 2
- nil – 1

Any patient with a GCS of 8 or less will have reduced airway reflexes and a high risk of aspiration. These patients, and those in whom the GCS falls by more than 2 points, should be referred to the ICU, if appropriate, as they will almost certainly require intubation.

In non-trauma patients who have been unconscious for 6 hours:

- 40% will have taken some form of sedative
- and of the remaining 60%

  - 40% have hypoxic brain injury (for example, following cardiac arrest)
  - 30% have a cerebrovascular cause (infarct or haemorrhage)
  - 25% have a metabolic coma.

Because hypoxic brain injury and stroke are by far the most common causes of non-traumatic coma, it is not surprising that 23% of these patients die within 1 hour, 64% within 1 week, 76% within 1 month, and 88% within 1 year.

Traumatic brain injury (TBI) is common and is the leading killer and cause of disability in children and young adults. Most research on brain injury and brain protection has been done in TBI but the principles are the same for all brain injury, whether caused by trauma or not.

There are many different causes of an unconscious patient and there is sometimes no history. A systematic approach is therefore required. Unconscious patients should always be considered an emergency. A, B, C, D, E is the system used to assess them:

- **A** – ensure patent, safe airway and treat if needed
- **B** – ensure adequate breathing and treat if needed
- **C** – assess circulation and treat if needed
- **D** – assess disability. The simple AVPU scale can be used at first, but the Glasgow Coma score should also be recorded so that any later changes can be documented precisely
- **E** – expose and examine the patient fully once A, B, and C is stable. Certain clusters of signs may point to a particular diagnosis
- While all this is going on, request a bedside glucose measurement.

Patients with focal neurological signs but no meningism are likely to have a stroke or tumour. Patients with meningism are likely to have meningitis or subarachnoid haemorrhage. Patients with neither focal signs nor meningism are likely to have hypoxic brain injury, intoxication, metabolic problems, severe sepsis, hypothermia, or epilepsy (non-convulsive status epilepticus is unusual, but one-fifth of patients with status may not appear to be convulsing).

The diagnosis and deliberation must not delay the need to actively treat A, B, C. In meningococcal meningitis securing the airway, and administering oxygen and intravenous fluid could save the patient's life more quickly than antibiotics (although in practice these are given together).

Indications for intubation in brain injury, if appropriate, are:

- coma (GCS 8 or less)
- loss of protective laryngeal reflexes from any cause
- ventilatory insufficiency (hypoxaemia or hypercapnia)
- spontaneous hyperventilation causing a low CO_2
- respiratory arrhythmia
- in certain situations where patients may need intubation prior to transfer (significantly deteriorating conscious level, bilateral fractured mandible, bleeding into the airway, or seizures).

Brain injury

Primary brain injury has limited treatment (it has already happened), so efforts have concentrated on preventing secondary brain injury. Secondary injury has a profound influence on outcome. It occurs as a result of the complications of primary brain injury – raised intracranial pressure, ischaemia, oedema and infection. It is important to realise that these complications are usually delayed and are therefore amenable to intervention. In TBI, the main precipitants of secondary injury are hypotension and hypoxaemia. Hypoxaemia, as defined by oxygen saturations < 90%, and hypotension, as defined by a systolic blood pressure of < 90 mmHg, are associated with a statistically significant worse outcome and are common at the scene of injury. Patients with severe TBI who are intubated in the prehospital setting have a better outcome.

Following brain injury, specific cells are rendered dysfunctional although not mechanically destroyed. If the subsequent environment is favourable, many of these cells can recover. Hypoxia or ischaemia can facilitate irreversible damage.

Cerebral blood flow

Cerebral blood flow (CBF) is around 15% cardiac output and is affected by various factors (Figure 9.1).

- A high $PaCO_2$ increases CBF by vasodilatation of blood vessels. Conversely, a low $PaCO_2$ causes vasoconstriction – reducing the $PaCO_2$ from 5 to 4 kPA (38·5–30·7 mmHg) reduces CBF by almost 30%.
- Hypoxaemia < 7·5 kPA (51·5 mmHg) has the effect of increasing CBF.
- Certain drugs affect CBF.

CBF is controlled by alterations in cerebral perfusion pressure (CPP) and cerebral vascular resistance (R). CBF = CPP/R. Cerebral perfusion pressure is the pressure gradient in the brain or the difference between the incoming arteries and the outgoing veins.

$$CPP = MAP - \text{venous pressure}$$

Venous pressure is equal to intracranial pressure (ICP), so CPP is usually expressed as:

$$CPP = MAP - ICP$$

Like the kidneys, the brain autoregulates blood flow so that it is constant between a MAP of 50 and 150 mmHg there is autoregulation (see Figure 9.1). CBF is regulated by changes in resistance of cerebral arteries. Unlike the rest of the body, the larger arteries play a main role in this. Local chemicals, endothelial mediators, and neurogenic factors are thought to be responsible. However, blood vessels in injured areas of the brain do not respond to normal regulation. Hypercapnia causes vasodilatation in normal tissue but diverts blood away from injured areas (the steal phenomenon). Hypocapnia may

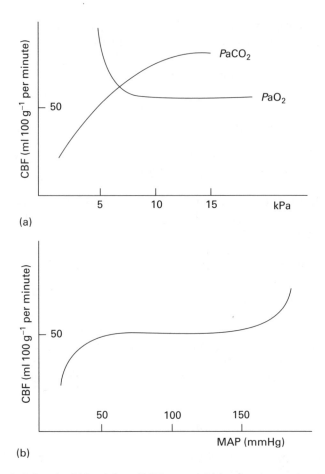

Figure 9.1 Cerebral blood flow (CBF), arterial blood gases and mean arterial pressure (MAP). (a) Between 3·5 and 10·6 kPa CO_2 there is an almost linear increase in CBF. There is little change in CBF until below 7·5 kPa O_2. (b) Autoregulation of cerebral perfusion occurs between a MAP of 60 and 150. Beyond these limits, CBF is dramatically affected

increase blood flow through damaged vessels leading to oedema (inverse steal).

The brain is uniquely vulnerable to secondary insults and less capable of maintaining an adequate blood flow and metabolic balance. A decrease in CBF in an injured brain may induce ischaemia; an increase in CBF may induce oedema.

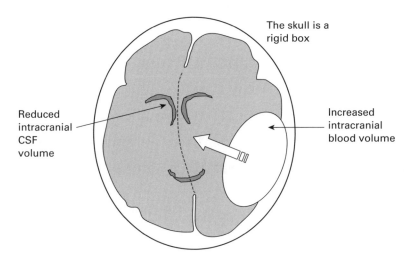

Figure 9.2 The Monro–Kellie doctrine. The CT scan shows a large extradural haematoma. Brainstem herniation eventually occurs

Raised intracranial pressure

Normal supine intracranial pressure is 7–17 mmHg and is frequently measured on neurointensive care units. Cerebral perfusion pressure can then be calculated and manipulated. A reasonable estimate of ICP can be made in patients with brain injury who are not sedated:

- drowsy and confused with GCS 13–15: ICP 20 mmHg
- GCS < 8: ICP 30 mmHg

Clinical features of raised ICP are nausea and vomiting, confusion and a reduced conscious level. Raised ICP can occur in cerebral haemorrhage, infarction with surrounding oedema, tumours, encephalitis, global ischaemia, or after TBI. As the skull is a rigid box, its contents are incompressible so ICP depends on the volume of intracranial contents (normally 5% blood, 5–10% CSF, and 85% brain). The Monro–Kellie doctrine is named after two Scottish anatomists (Figure 9.2). It states that, as the cranial cavity is a closed box, any change in intracranial blood volume is accompanied by an opposite change in CSF volume, if intracranial pressure is to be maintained.

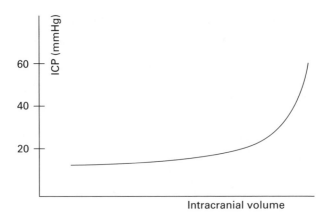

Figure 9.3 Effect of increasing intracranial volume on intracranial pressure (ICP)

When ICP is raised the following occurs:

- CSF moves into the spinal canal and there is increased reabsorption into the venous circulation;
- compensatory mechanisms are eventually overwhelmed, so further small changes in volume lead to large changes in pressure (Figure 9.3);
- as ICP rises further, CPP and CBF decrease;
- eventually brainstem herniation (coning) occurs.

The principles of brain protection

Preventing raised ICP and saving the penumbra (the area around the primary injury with potential to recover) with its compromised microcirculation is important. An uncontrolled increase in ICP and brainstem herniation is the major cause of death after TBI or primary brain haemorrhage. Because raised ICP can be caused by an increase in the volume of blood, CSF, or brain tissue, treatment is aimed at reducing the volume of these three components and is summarised in Table 9.1.

The cerebral metabolic rate for oxygen is the volume of oxygen utilised by the brain. It is around 50 ml per minute

Table 9.1 Methods to reduce intracranial pressure (ICP)

Blood	CSF	Brain tissue
Avoid high $PaCO_2$	Surgical drainage	Mannitol for generalised oedema
Nurse head up 15⁰ if possible		Steroids for tumour-related oedema
Avoid coughing and straining*		Frusemide also sometimes used
Keep head in midline*		

*To encourage venous drainage. CSF, cerebrospinal fluid.

and is reduced in hypothermia by 5% for each degree celsius drop. Hypothermia has been used in the past for cerebral protection during complex cardiac and neurosurgery. Interest in its potential as a treatment for brain injury has resurfaced. Animal models demonstrate its benefits but actively cooling normothermic humans with brain injury has not been shown to improve outcome. However, the converse applies. Pyrexia is associated with an adverse outcome in brain injury, including stroke, and should be treated. Active rewarming of patients who arrive with mild hypothermia in the early period after head injury is discouraged.

Hypertonic saline has been studied extensively in traumatic brain injury. The theory is that the hypertonic solution will draw intracellular water into the intravascular space, reducing cerebral oedema and expanding intravascular volume at the same time. The results of clinical trials have been mixed. In patients with other injuries, such as burns, there is an increased incidence of renal failure and death with the use of hypertonic saline, so its use is not recommended in the routine resuscitation of trauma victims.

Treatment protocols for traumatic brain injury that use the physiological principles outlined above improve outcome (Box 9.2). This is also true of non-traumatic conditions such as bacterial meningitis with raised intracranial pressure. Therefore the priority in managing all patients with brain injury, whether subarachnoid haemorrhage, TBI, meningitis with raised ICP, or stroke, is to prevent secondary brain injury.

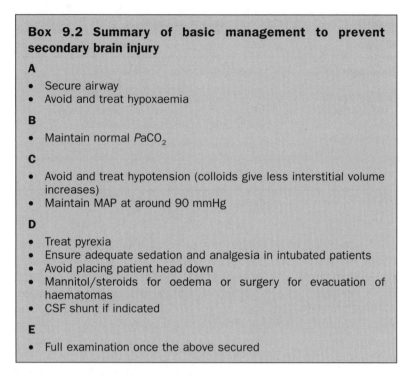

Box 9.2 Summary of basic management to prevent secondary brain injury

A

- Secure airway
- Avoid and treat hypoxaemia

B

- Maintain normal $PaCO_2$

C

- Avoid and treat hypotension (colloids give less interstitial volume increases)
- Maintain MAP at around 90 mmHg

D

- Treat pyrexia
- Ensure adequate sedation and analgesia in intubated patients
- Avoid placing patient head down
- Mannitol/steroids for oedema or surgery for evacuation of haematomas
- CSF shunt if indicated

E

- Full examination once the above secured

Subarachnoid haemorrhage

Subarachnoid haemorrhage (SAH) is included here as an example of brain injury because misdiagnosis is common. It occurs in 6–12 per 100 000 per year and has a peak incidence around the age of 50 years. Headache is common, but studies have found that, if patients with the worst headache of their lives and a normal neurological examination only were considered, 12% had SAH. Neurological examination is often normal and in these cases, a third of patients are misdiagnosed in studies. These studies also show that misdiagnosis leads to worse outcome – 65% misdiagnosed patients rebled and rebleeding carries a 40–50% mortality.

SAH commonly presents with a thunderclap headache – a distinct, sudden, severe headache. It need not be in any location; neck pain or vomiting may predominate. The first episode of severe headache cannot be classified as migraine or tension headache (International Headache Society). The sudden release of catecholamines can cause cardiac arrhythmias. Non-contrast CT scans are sensitive, but the pick-up rate decreases each day (92% on the same day, 76% 2 days later, and 58% 5 days later). MRI may be more sensitive in detecting SAH more than 4 days later. A negative CT scan does not exclude SAH. Lumbar puncture (LP) should then be performed (spectrophotometry to look for xanthochromia is most accurate. This is present within 4 hours, maximum at 1 week and persists for 3 weeks). The sample should be protected from light in transit and spun down immediately. SAH is suggested by ≥ 1000 red cells mm^{-3} but traumatic taps are common (20%). The method of counting red cells in tube 1 and 3 to distinguish a pathological from a traumatic tap can be unreliable. Since up to 6% people have incidental aneurysms, this is highly relevant. CSF pressure measurements should always be performed in diagnostic LPs.

Ultra-early rebleeding in SAH is not uncommon and this should justify immediate CT scanning followed by LP and transfer to the nearest neurosurgical centre. In one study, 17% patients had ultra-early rebleeding (admitted within 24 hours of bleed but rebled before surgery, which was scheduled for the next day). Ultra-early rebleeding was more likely to occur if it had happened once already, if systolic blood pressure was > 200 mmHg, and if the GCS was lower.

Most patients with SAH will be transferred to a neurosurgical centre for further treatment. Some of these patients will require intubation with anaesthesia and invasive monitoring prior to departure. Any fall in MAP during anaesthesia could reduce CPP to a critical level with a significant risk of adversely affecting outcome. Prognosis in SAH for those that reach hospital is that one-third will be in a coma, one-third will develop neurological deterioration, and one-third will make a good recovery.

Sedatives as a cause of coma – tricyclic poisoning

The most common sedative with potential for serious complications in the UK is tricyclic poisoning. This accounts for up to half of all adult admissions with poisoning to ICUs. It is the leading cause of death from drug overdose in patients who arrive in the Emergency Department alive. The typical cluster of signs includes coma within 1–2 hours of ingestion, respiratory depression, dilated pupils, divergent strabismus, myoclonic jerks, and bilateral upgoing plantars. A neutrophilia is commonly seen. Potentially lethal cardiovascular complications occur (arrhythmias and hypotension). The 12-lead ECG on admission can predict toxicity in that the majority of patients at risk for arrhythmias or convulsions will have a QRS width > 160 ms. Cardiotoxicity is due to slowing of the first phase of depolarisation through the His–Purkinje system and myocardium with a resulting prolongation of the QRS complex. The development of arrhythmias is made worse by a rapid heart rate, hypoxaemia from upper airway obstruction, acidosis, hypotension, and the anticholinergic effects of tricyclics. Although sinus tachycardia is more common (leading to problems differentiating this from ventricular tachycardia because of the wide QRS), bradyarrhythmias also occur owing to impaired cardiac automaticity. These are treated with temporary pacing, chronotropic drugs, or high dose intravenous glucagon. ECG changes are mainly due to sodium channel blockade and it is thought that sodium loading is one reason why sodium bicarbonate acts as an "antidote" to tricyclic poisoning. In the only human study reported, 91 patients with severe tricyclic poisoning were given sodium bicarbonate. Hypotension was corrected in 96% of patients, QRS prolongation in 80%, and conscious level in 47%. Current recommendations are that 50–100 ml boluses of 8·4% sodium bicarbonate are given when the QRS duration is > 120 ms, and there are malignant arrhythmias or hypotension (after securing the airway, giving oxygen, and administering fluid). Sodium bicarbonate is given even if there is no metabolic acidosis until the arterial pH is 7·4–7·5.

Imaging in coma

Recent advances in neuroimaging have increased our diagnostic ability. Computed tomography (CT) and magnetic resonance imaging (MRI) are the two techniques used in acutely ill adults. CT is the investigation of choice in trauma, subarachnoid haemorrhage, or stroke. It is readily available, quick and virtually all patients can be scanned. MRI provides images in several planes and provides superior grey/white matter contrast with a high sensitivity for most pathological processes compared with CT. MRI would be the investigation of choice in suspected posterior fossa lesions, epilepsy, and inflammatory processes. MRI is also more sensitive for thin extradural haematomas and diffuse axonal injury in trauma but requires special consideration for anaesthetised patients because of the interference from the electromagnetic field to anaesthetic and monitoring equipment.

Brain imaging is usually undertaken as soon as A, B, C are stable and a full evaluation has led to a differential diagnosis. When imaging is undertaken, it should lead to a diagnosis or have the potential to change management.

Brain injury following cardiac arrest

Cerebral ischaemia can be global (complete in cardiac arrest or incomplete in hypotension) or focal (as in cerebrovascular disease). In complete global ischaemia, waste products accumulate and the integrity of cell membranes breaks down, leaking potassium out of cells and allowing calcium into cells. Neurotransmitters accumulate and the chance of brain recovery is thought to be small after 4–5 minutes.

The widespread use of CPR often brings unrealistic expectations of recovery following cardiac arrest. Prognosis after cardiac arrest has been extensively investigated. A summary is as follows:

- In a Dutch study, survival to discharge of 8% for witnessed arrests at home and 18% outside the home was observed.
- In a German study, survival to discharge of 5·3–16·6% after out-of-hospital resuscitation was observed.
- A review of 26 000 in-hospital arrests showed 15·2% survival to discharge.
- Another study showed 8% survival to discharge after in-hospital cardiac arrest.
- 20–50% survivors have neurological or neuropsychological deficits.

These studies include all types of cardiorespiratory arrest, ranging from ventricular fibrillation on a Coronary Care Unit to cardiorespiratory arrest in multiple organ failure on the

ICU. The British Medical Association and UK Royal College of Nursing guidelines on "decisions related to cardiopulmonary resuscitation" make the following points and discuss in detail the principles surrounding communication, advance decision-making, and legal issues (see Further Reading below):

- Cardiorespiratory function ceases as part of dying, thus CPR can theoretically be attempted on every individual prior to death. So it is essential to identify patients in whom cardiorespiratory arrest is a terminal event in their illness and in whom CPR would be inappropriate
- It should be made clear that a "Do not attempt CPR" refers to CPR only. All other treatments will still be given unless specified to the contrary.
- In the UK, it is good practice to discuss with patients their wishes regarding CPR, if appropriate, but it is not mandatory.
- In cases of incapacity, the role of the next of kin in England and Wales is to communicate what the patient would have wanted in the circumstances. They have no legal jurisdiction and clinical decisions remain the responsibility of the specialist in charge of the patient's care.
- Good communication is the essential ingredient in decision-making on CPR.

Mini-tutorial: decision-making after cardiac arrest

Clinicians know that CPR has a poor outcome in most cases; communication around this point can be difficult. Therefore various investigators have attempted to predict outcome based on physiological observations post-arrest. One paper looked at predictors of death and neurological outcome in 130 out-of-hospital witnessed cardiac arrest survivors presenting to the Emergency Department. The investigators used time to return of spontaneous circulation, systolic blood pressure at the time of presentation, and a simple neurological examination to score patients (Table 9.2):

- return of spontaneous circulation < 25 minutes (score 0) or > 25 minutes (score 1)
- systolic BP at time of presentation > 90 mmHg (score 0) or < 90 mmHg (score 1)
- initial neurological examination: alert and orientated/rousable/ moves extremities (score 0) or unresponsive with only simple reflexes (score 1).

Table 9.2 Score after cardiac arrest and prognosis

Score	Mortality (%)	Neurological outcome (%)
0	19	85
1	45	58
2	63	29
3	94	0

The authors suggested that a simple scoring system could be used to triage patients and select those who would benefit from early aggressive measures such as urgent cardiac revascularisation. Note that pupil reflexes were not included in neurological examination – this is because the drugs used during CPR affect pupils, and pupillary reflexes should never be used as a prognostic sign immediately following cardiac arrest.

Although the above may be evidence to support decision-making, this is an incredibly difficult area as there is plenty of anecdotal evidence to show that some people survive to discharge against all the odds.

Self-assessment – case histories

1. A 20-year-old man is admitted unresponsive with a suspected heroin overdose. He received 400 micrograms intravenous naloxone in the Emergency Department and was sent up to the ward with a GCS of 15. You find him unresponsive, lying supine, and snoring loudly. He has an oxygen mask on and the pulse oximeter shows his oxygen saturations are 99%. His other vital signs are: blood pressure 110/60 mmHg, pulse 70 per minute, respiratory rate 5 per minute, temperature 37°C. How do you assess and manage him?

2. A 40-year-old man is found collapsed in his room with a bottle of tablets nearby. No history is available. On examination his airway is clear, breathing is normal, blood pressure is 80/40 mmHg, pulse is 130 per minute, sinus tachycardia with a broad QRS complex. He is unresponsive, has globally reduced tone, although he appears to have jerking movements every so often and has bilateral upgoing plantars with dilated pupils. What is your management?

3. A 25-year-old builder was hit on the head by machinery and is brought in unresponsive to the Emergency Department. There is a haematoma to the left side of his head. Airway is clear, breathing is normal, and he is cardiovascularly stable (blood pressure 140/70 mmHg and pulse 90 per minute). His Glasgow Coma Score is calculated as 7 out of 15. What is your management?

4. A 70-year-old man is brought in with a dense left hemiplegia. His blood pressure is 220/100 and pulse is 75, sinus rhythm. A colleague calls you to ask whether this blood pressure should be treated acutely and whether the patient has "malignant hypertension". Discuss your management.

5. A 30-year-old lady describes a sudden severe headache followed by vomiting. She has become drowsy on the way to hospital. You assess her GCS as 12. Outline your management priorities.

6. A 19-year-old man arrives having been found unresponsive by his girlfriend in the morning. He went to bed the evening before complaining of 'flu-like symptoms and a headache. On examination he has a GCS of 8, respiratory rate 30 per minute, pulse 130 per minute, BP 70/40 mmHg, SaO_2 98% on 10 litres per minute oxygen. There is some neck stiffness and a faint purpuric rash on his trunk. What is your management?

7. A 70-year-old lady is admitted having fallen off a step-ladder and injured her head. She has been lying on the floor for 4 hours. Her vital signs on admission are: GCS 4, respiratory rate 10 per minute, pulse 30 per minute, BP 60/30 mmHg, and temperature 29°C. Her arterial blood gases show: pH 7·20, $PaCO_2$ 6·0 kPA (46 mmHg), PaO_2 11·0 kPA (84·6 mmHg), bicarbonate 17·2 mmol/l, BE − 12. What is your management? What are your thoughts on the reasons for her abnormal vital signs?

8. A 23-year-old man arrives in the Emergency Department unconscious. He was the passenger in a car involved in a high-speed accident and was found by the paramedics, having been ejected from the car. He has extensive contusions on his head with a fixed and dilated right pupil. He groans and withdraws his limbs from painful stimuli on the right, but does not move his left side. He will not open his eyes. What is his GCS? What is his prognosis? Outline your management plan.

9. A 62-year-old man is resuscitated from a cardiac arrest. He had a pancreatoduodenectomy 3 days before for cancer. Twenty-four hours after the arrest he has a heart rate of 100 per minute, BP 118/75 mmHg, and a good urine output. Neurological examination reveals no pupillary light reflexes, no spontaneous or roving eye movements and absent motor reflexes. Discuss the neurological prognosis for this patient.

Self-assessment – discussion

1. In this case, the partially obstructed airway (snoring) should be relieved. The respiratory rate in this patient is 5 per minute. Oxygen saturation measurements do not assess ventilation. Arterial blood gas analysis will reveal a respiratory acidosis. Naloxone has a short half-life. This patient is unresponsive and requires either a naloxone infusion or intubation because of the risk of aspiration.

2. This case describes the characteristic cluster of signs seen in tricyclic poisoning and the label on the bottle of tablets found nearby will confirm this. The management starts with A (intubation), B, C (fluid), and D – including bedside glucose measurement and arterial blood gases as first line tests. Sinus tachycardia with a broad QRS complex and hypotension is common in serious tricyclic poisoning and can be difficult to distinguish from ventricular tachycardia. A 12-lead ECG may help to distinguish the two; 50 ml boluses of 8·4% sodium bicarbonate is given, even with a normal arterial pH, when the QRS duration is greater than 120 ms, if there are malignant arrhythmias or persistent hypotension (after securing the airway, and giving a high concentration of oxygen and intravenous fluid). CT scanning of the brain is not necessarily indicated when there is a clear history and signs consistent with poisoning.

3. The builder with a head injury should be managed by a team experienced in major trauma and ATLS (Advanced Trauma and Life Support) – this will ensure that other injuries are not missed. A (with cervical spine control), B, and C are still the immediate management in this case. Tracheal intubation is indicated and the anaesthetist will pay attention to preventing secondary brain injury by the following means:

- Even though the patient is unconscious, he will be given a general anaesthetic and paralysed before intubation to avoid any rise in intracranial pressure (tracheal intubation is extremely stimulating causing a rise in blood pressure and tachycardia in people not fully sedated).
- $PaCO_2$ will be kept within normal range and constantly monitored; hypoxaemia will be avoided.
- MAP will be maintained at around 90 mmHg (blood pressure not too high and not too low).
- The patient will be catheterised to avoid the stimulation of a full bladder, which may lead to a rise in ICP as well as increasing anaesthetic requirements.
- He will need an urgent CT scan of the head and neck, which may indicate the need for urgent neurosurgical intervention.

4. Hypertension following stroke is a common response to brain ischaemia. Blood pressure should not be lowered as blood supply to the potentially viable ischaemic penumbra could be compromised. Many stroke patients are normally hypertensive so a "normal" blood pressure may in fact be too low. The use of sublingual nifedipine gives an unpredictable response and may end up extending the stroke. If the stroke is caused by haemorrhage (in 15% cases), some neurologists would consider lowering an excessively high blood pressure in a controlled way, but not to "normal" levels – seek expert advice. In this patient, attention must be paid to the following: airway, oxygen

saturations, hydration, treatment of fever, lowering of high glucose levels, and good nursing care. "Malignant" hypertension is rare and the term "hypertensive crisis" is better. It occurs either on a background of hypertensive disease or as part of other conditions – eclampsia, phaeochromocytoma, and postoperatively (cardiac surgery). There is progressive severe hypertension with encephalopathy (confusion, headache, visual disturbances, fitting, reduced conscious level) and other end-organ damage: renal impairment and heart failure. If this occurs on a background of hypertensive disease, oral therapy is preferred as sudden dramatic falls in blood pressure may cause organ damage through hypoperfusion.

5. The history is consistent with subarachnoid haemorrhage. Management priorities here are to ensure a patent, protected airway and to administer oxygen. Assess and treat any breathing or circulation problems. This patient is drowsy. A formal GCS and neurological examination should be performed. This will provide an objective assessment of subarachnoid haemorrhage according to the World Federation of Neurological Surgeons scale (Table 9.3). A bedside glucose measurement is required. If A, B, C, and D are stable, there is time for a full history and examination. Arterial blood gas analysis would be helpful in assessing oxygenation, ventilation, and perfusion, all important in the prevention of secondary brain injury. The patient should be transferred for an urgent CT scan and neurosurgical opinion as soon as possible.

Table 9.3 World Federation of Neurological Surgeons SAH grading

WFNS grade	GCS	Major focal neurological deficit
1	15	Absent
2	13–14	Absent
3	13–14	Present
4	7–12	Present or absent
5	3–6	Present or absent

6. The most important diagnosis is meningococcal sepsis. However, immediate management priorities are A, B, C. The low GCS score indicates the need for urgent intubation. The patient requires fluid loading whilst preparations for intubation are made. A bedside glucose measurement and arterial blood gas is required. A full history and formal examination can be done once A, B, and C are stable. Blood cultures should be taken and intravenous antibiotics given whilst arrangements are made for an urgent CT of the head. Lumbar puncture is not necessary in cases of obvious meningococcal meningitis. Clotting abnormalities are a contraindication to LP. The bacteria can be

isolated from blood cultures and swabs of the throat and skin lesions. This patient requires further management on the ICU.

7. This lady has a head injury and an unstable cervical spine until proven otherwise. Intubation is indicated, with careful immobilisation of the C-spine. Intravenous atropine and warmed fluids are required to treat the circulation abnormalities. The arterial blood gases show a metabolic acidosis from hypoperfusion. Persistent hypotension may require invasive monitoring and vasoactive drugs. Active rewarming is indicated in severe hypothermia. A bedside glucose measurement and arterial blood gas are required. Differential diagnosis is straightforward hypothermia from lying on the floor or spinal shock. Spinal shock results from spinal cord concussion and gives rise to 24–72 hours of initial paralysis, hypotonicity, and areflexia. Return of activity below the level of the injury, such as the bulbocavernous reflex (anal sphincter contraction in response to tugging on the urinary catheter), signifies the end of spinal shock. Prolonged absence of distal motor function or perirectal sensation indicates complete spinal cord injury. Resuscitation in spinal shock includes raising the legs to reduce peripheral blood pooling, intravenous atropine to block vagal effects, vasopressors to support blood pressure, and high dose intravenous methylprednisolone, which improves outcome by minimising spinal oedema and by its anti-inflammatory actions. Once A, B, and C are stable, urgent CT imaging of the head and neck should be arranged with referral to the neurosurgical team if required.

8. The patient's GCS is 7 (E1, M4, V2). He has signs consistent with an extradural haematoma. These arise from tears in the dural arteries, usually the middle meningeal artery, and are often associated with linear skull fractures over the parietal or temporal areas. Extradural haematomas account for 1% of severe head injuries. The prognosis is generally good as the primary brain injury is usually not serious. However, secondary brain injury occurs rapidly owing to raised intracranial pressure, and is fatal if the clot is not evacuated. Immediate measures to reduce ICP may be required whilst surgery is being prepared. Extradural haematomata classically present as a loss of consciousness immediately after injury, followed by a lucid interval, and then a gradually decreasing conscious level associated with the development of an ipsilateral fixed dilated pupil and contralateral hemiparesis. However, presentation may be atypical or with coma, as in this case. Management in the Emergency Department is directed at stabilising life-threatening problems with A, B, or C, initiating measures to reduce intracranial pressure and transferring the patient safely to theatre. The only procedure to delay craniotomy would be life-threatening haemorrhage. It may be possible to perform a laparotomy and craniotomy simultaneously.

9. The patient has suffered global cerebral ischaemia following cardiac arrest. The best neurological recovery is seen in patients

who have a short duration of coma. Patients who remain in a coma 7–14 days after global ischaemia are unlikely to ever become independent. Individual signs suggesting neurological recovery are related to certain brainstem reflexes at the time of the initial examination. Absent light reflexes during the initial examination (allowing for the effects of cardiac arrest drugs to have worn off) place the patient in a very poor prognostic category. The presence of pupillary light reflexes with the return of spontaneous eye opening and conjugate eye movements, accompanied by motor responses, improves the prognosis and chance of independence. Based on this patient's examination at 24 hours, independent function is very unlikely.

Further reading

Eker C, Asgeirsson B, Grande P-O, Schalen W, Nordstrom C-H. Improved outcome after severe head injury with a new therapy based on principles for brain volume regulation and preserved microcirculation. *Crit Care Med* 1998;**11**:1881–6.

Hughes RAC, ed. *Neurological emergencies*. London: BMJ Books, 2000.

Levy DE, Bates D, Caronna JJ *et al.* Prognosis in non-traumatic coma. *Ann Intern Med* 1981;**94**:293–301.

Roberts I, Schierhout G, Alderson P *et al.* Absence of the evidence for the effectiveness of five interventions routinely used in the intensive care management of severe head injury: a systematic review. *J Neurol Neurosurg Psychiat* 1998;**65**:729–33.

Thompson RJ, McCullough PA, Kahn JK, O'Neill WW. Prediction of death and neurologic outcome in the Emergency Department in out-of-hospital cardiac arrest survivors. *Am J Cardiol* 1998;**81**:17–21.

http://www.bma.org.uk/ap.nsf/Content/cardioresus

10: Optimising physiology before surgery

By the end of this chapter you will be able to:

- understand the nature of the medical consultation
- assess perioperative risk in patients with cardiac and respiratory disease
- understand the principles behind 'preoptimisation'
- prepare a patient for emergency surgery
- apply this to your clinical practice

The medical consultation

The physician is part of a team (including the surgeon, anaesthetist, nurse, and physiotherapist) whose role is to plan perioperative care. This involves postoperative care as well as preoperative care. The physician's role is particularly in assessing the level of risk and recommending measures to reduce that risk, in consultation with the patient and colleagues. It is not his or her role to clear the patient for surgery, which implies no risk at all. Most requests are specifically to help the anaesthetist in the assessment of perioperative risk with particular attention being paid to cardiac and respiratory disease.

Physiological reserve is an important concept in patients facing major or emergency surgery and in critical illness generally. The cardiovascular system in particular has to mount a compensatory response to the physiological stress. Patients who lack the ability to do this because of impaired organ function have increased mortality as demonstrated by the American Society of Anaesthesiologists' classification of disease severity (Box 10.1).

Key components of the medical consultation are to:

- Find out the severity and stability of the disease in question.
- Specifically recommend measures to treat the disease, optimise the patient's function and reduce perioperative risk.
- Plan postoperative care with colleagues.

Box 10.1 ASA classification of disease severity (mortality increases with class)

ASA 1 Healthy patient

ASA 2 Mild systemic disease that does not limit function

ASA 3 Moderate systemic disease that limits function

ASA 4 Severe systemic disease that is a constant threat to life

ASA 5 Moribund patient who will not survive 24 hours without surgery

ASA 3E would indicate a patient who is ASA 3 undergoing emergency surgery. The ASA (American Society of Anesthesiologists) system does not account for age, smoking, or obesity, factors that also increase risk.

The assessment of patients with cardiac disease

The largest single cause of perioperative death is cardiac related. Cardiovascular disease affects 25% of the US population. Much work has been done to try to assess cardiovascular risk before surgery as perioperative myocardial infarction carries a 30–50% mortality. There are five main types of cardiac disease that present before surgery:

- ischaemic heart disease
- heart failure
- valvular disease
- cardiac arrhythmias especially atrial fibrillation
- hypertension.

The greater the cardiovascular stress during surgery, the greater the risk of cardiac complications (Table 10.1).

Ischaemic heart disease

Major clinical predictors of perioperative cardiac complications are patients with recent (within 6 months) myocardial infarction, severe or unstable angina, and significant arrhythmias. However, many patients have

Table 10.1 Risk of major perioperative cardiac event according to type of surgery

Low risk (< 1%)	Intermediate risk (1–5%)	High risk (> 5%)
Endoscopic procedures	Carotid endarterectomy	Emergency major surgery
Superficial procedures	Head & neck	Aortic/major vascular surgery
Cataract	Intraperitoneal	Peripheral vascular
Breast	Intrathoracic	Prolonged procedure with large fluid shifts/blood loss
	Orthopaedic	
	Prostate	

Table 10.2 Risk of major perioperative cardiac event according to type of patient

Minor	Intermediate	Major
Advanced age	Mild angina (class 1–2)	Unstable coronary syndromes • recent MI (< one month) • unstable/severe angina
Abnormal ECG	Previous myocardial infarction (history or ECG)	Decompensated heart failure
Rhythm other than sinus	Compensated or previous heart failure	Significant arrhythmias
Low functional capacity	Diabetes	Severe valve disease
History of stroke		
Uncontrolled hypertension		

controlled ischaemic heart disease and, although there are a number of tests available to assess this group, they are not necessarily helpful. History, examination, and resting ECG can readily categorise risk (Table 10.2).

Additional scoring systems have been developed (for example, the Goldman cardiac risk index) that can help quantify risk and these are based on observational studies. Probably the most useful measure with regard to ischaemic heart disease is the patient's functional ability. Risk is increased in patients who cannot reach 4 METS (metabolic equivalents) workload; 1 MET is equivalent to the oxygen consumption of a resting 40-year-old 70 kg man. Climbing a flight of stairs, briskly walking on the flat, mowing the lawn, swimming, or playing a round of golf is at least 4 METS.

Surgery may proceed without further evaluation in patients with minor risk factors and good function who are undergoing low or intermediate risk surgery. Patients with intermediate risk factors and poor functional capacity may need further evaluation and optimisation before surgery. Exercise ECG testing is widely available but impractical for many high risk surgical patients.

Dobutamine stress echocardiography is the best test to predict perioperative events, according to most studies. It has a 100% negative predictive value and patients with extensive ischaemia experience 10 times more perioperative cardiac events than those with limited ischaemia. Coronary angiography is indicated in appropriate high risk patients or intermediate risk patients after screening.

Overall, less than 10% surgery is associated with a perioperative cardiac event. However, vascular surgery poses particular risks because many of the risk factors for peripheral vascular disease are the same for coronary artery disease (diabetes, smoking, and hyperlipidaemia). In one study, 1000 consecutive patients with peripheral vascular disease but no clinical evidence of ischaemic heart disease underwent coronary angiography; 37% had at least one coronary artery stenosis of > 70%. The incidence is higher in vascular patients with clinical evidence of ischaemic heart disease – approximately 60%. Cardiac symptoms may be masked in some of these patients because their mobility is limited. Major vascular surgery is also associated with fluctuations in intravascular volume and blood pressure, which stress the heart.

Several randomised trials have looked at medical therapy to reduce perioperative risk (β blockers, nitrates and calcium channel blockers). There is evidence to suggest that perioperative β blockers reduce cardiac complications (ischaemic episodes, myocardial infarction, and mortality). One randomised trial used prophylactic atenolol immediately before and up to 7 days after non-cardiac surgery. This reduced the cardiovascular mortality rate at 6, 12, and 24 months. In both vascular and general surgery, atenolol reduces perioperative cardiac mortality and ischaemic complications. In a study on vascular patients, cardiac mortality and morbidity was reduced by bisoprolol from 34% to 3·4%. β blockers are therefore recommended for high risk patients and patients with hypertension, ischaemic heart disease, or risk factors for ischaemic heart disease. If preoperative administration is not possible, intravenous β blocker given at induction of anaesthesia followed by postoperative treatment is also effective. The intraoperative use of nitroglycerine in high risk patients does not affect outcome despite reduced ischaemia on the ECG.

The diagnosis of myocardial infarction in the perioperative period can be difficult. One half of patients do not have typical chest pain. They may present with arrhythmias, pulmonary oedema, hypotension, or confusion. ECG changes are common postoperatively and do not necessarily indicate myocardial infarction. Up to 20% postoperative patients have new ECG abnormalities – usually T wave changes. Creatinine kinase rises non-specifically with surgery and troponin measurements are more appropriate.

Heart failure

Lack of cardiopulmonary reserve is a more important predictor of perioperative death than cardiac ischaemia. It has long been observed that high risk patients who survive surgery have greater compensatory increases in cardiovascular and oxygen transport measurements than patients who die – non-survivors are unable to compensate for the added metabolic and cardiorespiratory demands of surgery and die of multiple organ failure. High risk patients are those who are most critically ill at the time of surgery or who face major surgery.

In the preoperative period, high risk patients have an increased incidence of severe physiological impairment as measured by a PA catheter. In many patients the baseline values can be improved by relatively simple measures, for example giving fluid or inotropes. Previous studies have shown that careful invasive monitoring of high risk patients in the perioperative period improves outcome. More recently, "preoptimisation" or screening to see which patients could benefit from giving therapy preoperatively has also been shown to improve outcome.

In one study, patients underwent preoperative invasive cardiovascular monitoring with a PA catheter and were classified as groups 1 (normal) to 4 (severe physiological impairment). All of group 1 survived surgery. Groups 2 and 3 had moderate physiological impairment, which could be corrected with simple measures. Their mortality was 8·5%. In group 4, with uncorrectable physiological impairment, seven patients had lesser surgery and survived, 19 were cancelled, and all 8 who went ahead with the planned surgery died. In another study, patients were divided in to three groups. Group 1 was assessed using a PA catheter and treated with fluid loading, afterload reduction, and/or inotropes 12 hours preoperatively. Group 2 was investigated and treated 3 hours preoperatively, and group 3 was the control (no PA catheter). The aim was to achieve a PAOP of 8–15 mmHg, cardiac index > 2·8 litres per minute m^{-2}, and SVR < 1100 dyn.s cm^{-5}. Patients with a PA catheter and subsequent intervention had significantly fewer adverse intraoperative events and less overall mortality.

Based on studies like this, practice is moving in the direction of invasive cardiac monitoring in high risk patients before major surgery in order to correct pre-existing physiological impairment and to improve compensatory responses. This illustrates the general importance of adequate resuscitation before major surgery.

Echocardiography does not appear to be a useful predictor of perioperative cardiac events, although a reduced ejection fraction correlates with an increased risk of perioperative pulmonary oedema.

Valvular heart disease

Severe aortic stenosis (AS) poses the greatest perioperative risk. This is because, if hypotension occurs during anaesthesia and surgery, it can be a difficult problem to correct. AS is a fixed obstruction and limits maximum cardiac output during stress. Patients cannot respond normally to the peripheral dilation associated with anaesthesia and blood pressure can fall dramatically. This causes myocardial ischaemia, as the myocardial hypertrophy seen in AS is associated with increased oxygen demand. AS may be asymptomatic and patients with severe stenosis do not necessarily exhibit classical features on examination. According to the Helsinki Ageing Study, 3% people aged 75–85 have critical aortic stenosis.

It is also important to recognise mitral stenosis because it is necessary to control the heart rate in order to preserve diastole. This aids filling of the left atrium and generates enough pressure to squeeze blood through the stenosed valve. The presence of any murmur requires a preoperative echocardiogram, and antibiotic prophylaxis is required for most patients with valve disease undergoing surgery.

Cardiac arrhythmias especially atrial fibrillation

Arrhythmias following surgery are common, often exacerbated by the abrupt withdrawal of cardiac drugs due to fasting. They are also caused by hypotension, metabolic derangements, and hypoxaemia – all of which are preventable. It is important that patients with heart disease are maintained on their usual drugs, via alternative routes if possible, during the perioperative period. This particularly applies to β blockers, which should be administered on the day of surgery.

Five per cent patients over the age of 65 have chronic atrial fibrillation (AF) and it is a common preoperative finding. Certain procedures are associated with the development of AF, for example intrathoracic surgery. Patients with chronic lung or cardiac disease are at greater risk of developing postoperative AF. The main difference in the preoperative period is that β- or calcium channel blockers are considered more effective than digoxin in controlling the ventricular rate during stress. If the patient is anticoagulated, this also needs to be addressed in the preoperative period.

Prophylactic cardiac pacing may be required prior to surgery in patients at risk of developing complete heart block. These include patients with bi- or trifascicular block on the ECG, and they should be assessed by a cardiologist.

Hypertension

The risks of preoperative hypertension are unclear, with some studies showing increased cardiovascular complications and others no increased risk. Hypertension alone is therefore considered a borderline risk factor. However, hypertension is a risk factor for ischaemic heart disease.

Mini-tutorial: preoptimisation of the high risk surgical patient

High risk surgical patients are those with poor preoperative status or who are about to undergo a major procedure or one involving heavy blood loss. In 1979, Shoemaker *et al.* defined the criteria for high surgical risk:

- patient history: age > 70 years with major limitations of physiological function, previous severe cardiopulmonary or vascular disease, severe nutritional disorders
- critical factors: severe multiple trauma, massive acute blood loss, shock, severe sepsis, respiratory failure, acute abdominal catastrophe, acute intestinal or renal failure
- surgical procedure: extensive surgery for cancer or prolonged surgery.

Shoemaker's group observed a mortality of 25% in their own high risk surgical patients. Outcome was dramatically influenced by the ability of the patient's cardiopulmonary system to adapt. Values for CO, DO_2, and oxygen uptake were significantly higher in survivors than in non-survivors. It was postulated that the observed increase in CO and DO_2 were circulatory responses owing to increased postoperative oxygen demand. However, subsequent trials which aimed for "supranormal" values in CO and DO_2 were associated with adverse outcomes.

In high risk surgical patients, reduced cardiac output may compromise perfusion in organs such as the gastrointestinal tract and kidney, leading to ischaemia and reperfusion injury. The subsequent release of reactive oxygen species and inflammatory mediators leads to activation of immune cells and distant organ injury (for example, lung and liver) leading to MODS. Early detection of gastrointestinal hypoperfusion could provide advance warning of this – it is associated with more severe organ dysfunction, longer ICU stay, and greater mortality in surgical and trauma patients. Gastrointestinal hypoperfusion as detected by gastric pH measurements (tonometry) in postoperative cardiac surgery patients has been shown to be an early indicator of circulatory failure and increased morbidity.

The role of dopexamine

In one randomised trial, Boyd *et al.* used dopexamine to increase perioperative DO_2 in high risk surgical patients. The mean dose of

---

dopexamine infused was 1·2 µg kg^{-1} per minute preoperatively and 1·3 µg kg^{-1} per minute postoperatively. Mortality at 28 days was 5·7% in the dopexamine group and 22·2% in the controls. A few years later, Wilson et al. randomised high risk patients into three groups. Controls received routine perioperative care and two groups were preoptimised. Optimisation consisted of invasive haemodynamic monitoring, fluid loading to achieve a PAOP of 12 mmHg, blood transfusion to achieve an Hb of > 11 g dl^{-1}, oxygen therapy to achieve saturations of > 94%, and either adrenaline or dopexamine to increase DO_2 to > 600 ml O_2 per minute. Inotropic support was continued during surgery and for at least 12 hours afterwards; 70% of patients had more than two Shoemaker entry criteria. Mortality was reduced in both the adrenaline and dopexamine groups (2% and 4%) compared with the controls (17%). This was statistically significant. Dopexamine also significantly reduced postoperative morbidity when compared with both the adrenaline and the control groups.

Dopexamine has anti-inflammatory properties as well as improving regional blood flow and renal function in rat models of sepsis to a greater extent than either dopamine or dobutamine. Its various anti-inflammatory effects have yet to be proved in clinical practice.

In most of these outcome studies, PA catheters were used to monitor cardiac output and calculate oxygen transport. Research has concentrated on developing and evaluating less invasive methods for assessing the adequacy of resuscitation. Intramucosal pH (pHi) has been shown to be of greater value in monitoring trauma patients than oxygen transport measurements. In elderly patients with proximal femur fractures, using oesophageal Doppler monitoring to guide volume replacement, led to more fluid administration to the treatment group and a significant reduction in hospital stay. There was no impact on hospital mortality, possibly because of the small numbers studied. In elective cardiac surgical patients with ejection fractions > 50%, patients who received volume expansion to maximum stroke volume had a significantly reduced morbidity and hospital stay. These studies support the concept that adequate fluid resuscitation is of vital importance in high risk surgical patients.

The assessment of patients with lung disease

Preoperative lung function tests and arterial blood gases can predict the need for postoperative ventilatory support and quantify the type and degree of respiratory impairment. High risk patients include those who are breathless at rest, have a

PaCO$_2$ > 6·0 kPa (46 mmHg), FEV1 > 1 litre, or an FEV1/FVC ratio of < 50%. Other factors which make pulmonary complications more likely include:

- upper abdominal or thoracic surgery (closer to the diaphragm carries higher risk)
- high ASA class
- COPD
- smoking within the previous 8 weeks
- surgery of longer than 3 hours duration
- obesity.

Certain measures may help to reduce perioperative pulmonary complications. These are: stopping smoking, preoperative inhaled β-agonists for patients with COPD, or intravenous steroids if needed, the use of regional anaesthesia (with or without general anaesthesia), and lung expansion exercises postoperatively. Morbidly obese patients (> 115 kg or 250 lb) and smokers are twice as likely to develop postoperative pneumonia.

Assessment of patients with other problems may be required. Impairment of any organ system leads to an increase in perioperative complications. Endocrine disorders (for example, diabetes), renal failure, liver disease, haematological, and neurological disorders are not discussed here. Other scoring systems have been developed that assist in the assessment of risk prior to surgery, for example the Child–Pugh classification of liver disease.

Preparation of patients prior to emergency surgery

Surgery, especially emergency surgery, is a physiological insult. In some cases surgery takes precedence over full resuscitation (for example, in ruptured aortic aneurysm), but in most cases there is time to resuscitate the patient. General and spinal anaesthesia sometimes involve a drop in blood pressure owing to vasodilatation, and this is exaggerated if the patient is volume-depleted prior to induction. Hypovolaemia before emergency surgery is common and is due to:

- vomiting and diarrhoea
- fasting
- bleeding
- fluid loss in to an obstructed bowel
- sepsis or SIRS.

As stated throughout this book, proper resuscitation makes a big difference to outcome – not only in terms of perioperative mortality but also in terms of postoperative morbidity. In terms of simple physiology (A, B, C) one should aim to restore the observations as far towards the patient's normal as possible before surgery. This is so that they can mount a successful compensatory response during the perioperative period.

Preoperative aims are:

- airway secure
- respiratory rate 10–30
- $PaO_2 > 10$ kPa (77 mmHg)
- well perfused with good cardiac output
- urine output > 1 ml kg^{-1} per hour
- haemoglobin > 8 g dl^{-1}
- normal electrolytes (especially K^+ and Mg_2^+)
- acceptable BE $(> - 5)$

Self assessment – case histories

1. A 75-year-old woman has been admitted 24 hours previously with large bowel obstruction. She is warm and tachycardic and had been unwell at home for several days before coming to hospital. Her urine output per hour has slowly decreased throughout the day and is now < 0.5 ml kg^{-1} per hour. She is scheduled for theatre in a few hours. Outline your management.

2. A 70-year-old woman is due for a partial gastrectomy for stomach cancer but the surgeons have noted that her ECG has changed in the last 4 weeks. There is new T wave inversion in leads V1–V4. You are asked to decide whether or not she has had a myocardial infarction. She says she had an hour of chest discomfort 2 weeks ago, but did not seek medical attention. She does not suffer from angina or breathlessness, and is walking around the hospital with no symptoms. What is her perioperative risk, what can you do to reduce that risk, and what do you advise the surgeons?

3. A 60-year-old man comes to the Outpatient Department, referred by an orthopaedic surgeon. The patient has a history of ischaemic heart disease and has had a myocardial infarction many years ago. He does not have angina nowadays (on treatment). He arrives using a walking stick because of his painful knee, which is due to be replaced. The orthopaedic surgeon has asked whether it is safe to proceed with the planned surgery in view of his heart disease. What is the question you are being asked? How do you assess the patient?

4. A 75-year-old lady is admitted following a fall and a fractured left neck of femur. There is no past medical history. She has been lying on the floor for 18 hours at home. On examination her skin feels warm and dry. She has the following vital signs: in pain, pulse 110/minute, BP 110/60 mmHg, RR 26 per minute, temperature 38°C, SaO_2 94% on air, urine output – has not passed urine since admission (not catheterised). There are coarse crackles at the left base of the lungs and a chest x ray film shows pneumonia. She is scheduled for theatre as soon as possible. What do you need to do before then?

5. You are asked to see a 60-year-old man who is being booked for an elective inguinal hernia repair. In the Outpatient Clinic it is noted that his oxygen saturations are 89% on air and he is breathless on exertion. You are asked to advise on his chest condition before surgery. Further history reveals that he is a lifelong smoker and used to be a miner. He has several years' history of breathlessness on exertion but has never seen a doctor about it. On examination he has hyperexpanded lungs and prolonged expiration with scattered wheeze. His chest x ray film shows clear lung fields and his arterial blood gases on air show: pH 7·4, $PaCO_2$ 6·0 kPa (46 mmHg), bicarbonate 27 mmol/l, BE + 1, PaO_2 7·5 kPa (57·6 mmHg). What is your advice to the surgeons?

6. A 65-year-old lady is admitted with small bowel obstruction, which is being treated with a nasogastric tube and intravenous fluids. She has a history of stable angina and hypertension. Her usual medication includes atenolol 50 mg a day. You are asked to see her urgently because her pulse is 140 per minute (previously 60 per minute). The ECG shows atrial fibrillation. Why has this happened and what is your management?

7. A 60-year-old man on treatment for angina and heart failure is admitted with bowel obstruction. He has been unwell with vomiting for 4 days. On examination he has a pulse of 100 per minute, BP 100/50 mmHg, RR 24 per minute, temperature 37·5°C and SaO_2 95% on air. His blood results show a raised white cell count and urea of 15 mmol litre^{-1} (BUN 41 mg dl^{-1}), creatinine 300 μmol litre^{-1} (3·6 mg dl^{-1}). His urea and creatinine were normal 3 months ago. He is scheduled for theatre as soon as possible. Should he be "preoptimised"?

Self assessment – discussion

1. Looking back, preoperative aims were summarised as:

    - airway secure
    - respiratory rate 10–30
    - $PaO_2 > 10$ kPa (77 mmHg)
    - well perfused with good cardiac output
    - urine output > 1 ml kg^{-1} per hour
    - haemoglobin > 8 g dl^{-1}
    - normal electrolytes (especially K^+ and Mg_2^+)
    - acceptable BE (> -5)

    Is this case due to simple hypovolaemia or is this patient developing SIRS? Management consists of A (giving a high concentration of oxygen), B (treating any breathing problems), and C (giving fluid). Hypoperfusion should be assessed further by measuring blood pressure, respiratory rate, skin temperature, and arterial blood gases. Invasive monitoring may be helpful. Particular attention should be paid to the possibility of electrolyte disturbances from nasogastric losses. Surgery should be postponed for a short time while resuscitation takes place – ask whether she should be preoptimised in a high dependency area.

2. Myocardial infarction is diagnosed from history, electrocardiogram changes, and a cardiac enzyme rise. Two out of three indicates a probable recent myocardial infarction. This, and the type of surgery, places the patient at high risk of perioperative cardiac complications but, as the surgery is for cancer, it would be impractical to postpone this for 6 months. In terms of function the patient is quite good with no angina, breathlessness, nor limitation of mobility. Post-myocardial infarction treatment is indicated (including a β blocker, which will also reduce perioperative risk). A discussion of the risks involved should take place between the surgeon, anaesthetist, and patient. High risk patient and high risk surgery should lead to consideration of perioperative invasive cardiac monitoring.

3. The questions being asked are:

    - How significant is this patient's ischaemic heart disease?
    - What is his perioperative cardiac risk?
    - Can that risk be reduced by any specific measures?

    The patient should be asked about cardiac symptoms and general function. The Goldman score can be used at this point. General cardiovascular risk factors should be sought and treated (for example, hypertension, high cholesterol, diabetes, and smoking). Perioperative β blockers would be indicated. He is an intermediate risk patient facing intermediate risk surgery with good function. However, his mobility may be limited by his painful knee, masking angina symptoms. Non-invasive cardiac testing may therefore be indicated to assess this further.

4. With the list of preoperative aims in Question 1 in mind, this patient needs oxygen therapy, treatment for pneumonia, and fluid for dehydration. Analgesia is required, but not with NSAIDs (oliguria). A urinary catheter and arterial blood gases are indicated. Blood should be sent for full blood count and electrolytes. In this case creatinine kinase levels should be measured, as the patient has been lying on the floor for a long time and has oliguria (possible rhabdomyolysis). Outcome is better after a fractured neck of femur if surgery is within 24 hours and regional anaesthesia is used. The dilemma here is that delaying surgery while waiting for the chest to improve may not help. Early surgery, good postoperative care, physiotherapy, and mobilisation may in fact be better for the chest.

5. This man has a new diagnosis of COPD. This can be confirmed by pulmonary function tests. He needs treatment for this condition under the supervision of a chest specialist. Once this is done and the patient is as fit as he can be (which may mean he is still breathless and hypoxaemic), the following recommendations should be made:

   - the patient should stop smoking
   - perioperative inhaled beta agonists should be prescribed.

   Intravenous steroids can be considered. Early mobilisation and chest physiotherapy are indicated after surgery and a discussion should take place with the anaesthetist and surgeon as to whether or not a general anaesthetic can be avoided.

6. The abrupt withdrawal of this patient's β blocker and possible electrolyte disturbance (from bowel obstruction and intravenous fluid administration) have caused atrial fibrillation in this lady with ischaemic heart disease. Treatment still starts with A, B, C. Correction of any low potassium or magnesium and intravenous administration of a β blocker is a logical course of action in this case.

7. Yes! This patient has significant premorbid conditions and is about to undergo major surgery. He already has symptoms and signs of organ dysfunction. Volume depletion may be the cause of his acute renal failure. He requires aggressive but careful fluid resuscitation in order to maximise his compensatory responses to surgery. He should be referred to the ICU where fluid therapy can be titrated using more advanced forms of monitoring. "Goal-directed therapy" in this patient may stop the slide from SIRS to MODS. Goals should be set according to the monitoring available in your hospital (pressure-based or flow-based). Useful tests to monitor the success or failure of resuscitation are clinical status

and biochemical markers of hypoperfusion (base deficit, lactate, and pHi). Inotropes should be commenced if appropriate. Dopexamine at a rate of 0·5–1·5 µg kg⁻¹ per minute can improve oxygen delivery and tissue perfusion. Monitoring should be continued during surgery and the immediate postoperative period. "Optimisation" after surgery is less effective in improving outcome.

Further reading

American College of Cardiology practice guidelines: perioperative cardiovascular evaluation for non-cardiac surgery. www.acc.org/clinical/statements.htm.

Berlauk JF, Abrams JH, Gilmour IJ, O'Connor SR, Knighton DR, Cerra FB *et al*. Pre-operative optimisation of cardiovascular haemodynamics improves outcome in peripheral vascular surgery. *Ann Surg* 1991;**214**:289–97.

Boyd O, Grounds RM, Bennett ED. A randomised clinical trial of the effect of deliberate peri-operative increase in oxygen delivery on mortality in high-risk surgical patients. *JAMA* 1993;**270**:2699–707.

Chassot P-G, Delabays A, Spahn DR. Pre-operative evaluation of patients with, or at risk of, coronary artery disease undergoing non-cardiac surgery. *Br J Anaesth* 2002;**89**:747–59.

Del Guercio L, Cohn J. Monitoring operative risk in the elderly. *JAMA* 1980;**243**:1350–5.

Goldman L, Caldera DL, Nussbaum SR *et al*. Multifactorial index of cardiac risk in non-cardiac surgical procedures. *New Engl J Med* 1977; **297**:845.

Juste RN, Lawson AD, Soni N. Minimising cardiac anaesthetic risk: the tortoise or the hare? *Anaesthesia* 1996;**51**:255–62.

Shoemaker WC, Czer LS. Evaluation of the biologic importance of various haemodynamic and oxygen transport variables: which variables should be monitored in post-operative shock? *Crit Care Med* 1979;**7**:424–31.

Sinclair S, James S, Singer M. Intra-operative intravascular volume optimisation and length of hospital stay after repair of proximal femur fractures: a randomised control trial. *BMJ* 1997;**315**:909–12.

Wilson J, Woods I, Fawcett J *et al*. Reducing the risk of major elective surgery: randomised control trial of pre-operative optimisation of oxygen delivery. *BMJ* 1999;**318**:1099–103.

http://www.acc.org/clinical/statements.htm

Index

Entries in **bold** refer to figures, those in *italics* refer to tables/boxed material